FORTY PLUS

FORTY PLUS

Use it, or lose it!
THE _ultimate_ FITNESS GUIDE

Andy Ripley & Dr Liz Ferris

STANLEY PAUL

LONDON · SYDNEY · AUCKLAND · JOHANNESBURG

For Sophie

Acknowledgements

I should like to thank the following for all their help and support during the preparation of this book: Sophie for her inspiration, Jules for his encouragement, Sarah for her patience and Dr Craig Sharp of the British Olympic Medical Centre for his expert guidance and advice.

Liz Ferris, 1991

Photograph Acknowledgements

Thanks are due to the following for allowing use of copyright photographs: ACE, AllSport, BBC, Colorsport, Liz Ferris, Matthew Ford, The Image Bank, Naomi James, Mail Newspapers, Mike Nicholson, Photo Source, Press Association, Chris Ralston, Andy Ripley

Contents

ONE

PART ONE · SETTING THE TARGETS

Opening New Doors

When Liz's daughter, Sophie, was ten, she painted a picture which was proudly framed by her mum and dad and hung in a place of parental honour (in the kitchen next to the paper-towel dispenser, above the sink). Liz says it is a constant source of inspiration. The picture shows two tables. On one table are things perceived by a ten-year-old to be kind to your body – fruit, natural juices, boots for walking, a radio. On the other are alcohol, slippers, a hamburger and a television. One table leads to a coffin. The other table leads to someone dancing at the end of a sunbeam.

Whatever your age or ability you can choose how you want to lead your life. As you become older, you may have fewer physical options. There are benefits that come with age – experience, memories, judgement, established friendships, a decreasing need to chase rainbows, material and emotional stability – but physically it's downhill from your late twenties onwards. But you can slow down the ageing process – if you choose to do so.

This book *isn't* about turning you into an Olympic high diver or an international rugby player. Nor do we want you to become obsessed with diet or exercise. We want *you* to think about making choices which can influence your well-being.

First, Liz and I will tell you about our own backgrounds, our experience of exercise and its beneficial effects. After revealing the changes ageing brings, Liz will guide you through the physical and psychological choices you have:

* stress and relaxation

* smoking or non-smoking

* training and competition

* drinking

* active or sedentary lifestyle

Then a number of famous Forty-somethings tell us how *they* have come to terms with the physical limitations of ageing. Finally, we have each set ourselves targets. My goal was to take up five new sporting activities, and Liz's goal was to take part in a short-course triathlon (swim-bike-run).

It's true that there are some things we can't change, and it's easy to make excuses – 'I'm the wrong size/shape,' 'I'm too old,' 'I can't afford it.' But there are *always*, however limited, choices you *can* make. We hope we can open a few doors for you – doors you may not have thought of opening before.

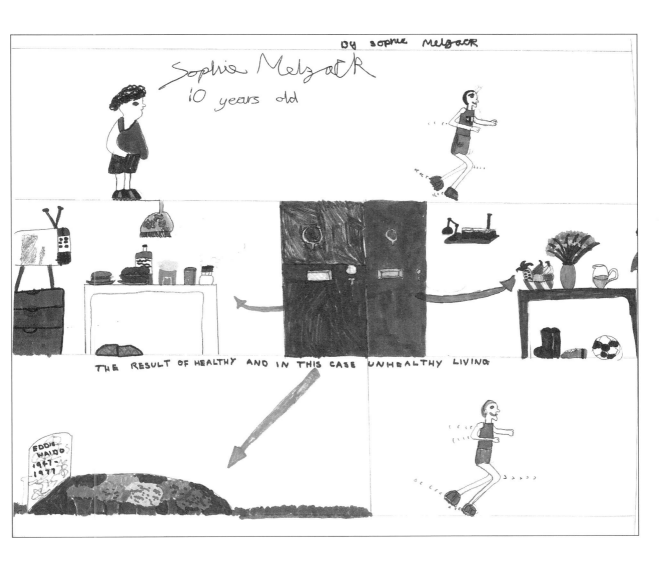

TWO

The Plans Take Shape

Liz's story

I have kept fit since I stopped diving in 1964. Recently, aged forty-eight, I did a treadmill exercise test at the British Olympic Medical Centre and discovered, to my glee, that I had the aerobic capacity of the average twenty-five-year-old woman. I tripped out of there skipping on air. All those years dancing on the end of a pin had not been wasted. Time and my genes have been good to me.

Physical challenges were introduced early in my family, although neither of my parents was involved in sport. When I was three, I entered the water for the first time and took to it like the proverbial duckling. At about the same time, I was detailed to run errands to the corner shop; a packet of sugar grew into a carrier bag full of groceries. Undaunted and eager to please, I would half-carry, half-drag this huge load home, enormously pleased with myself. My mother had her critics for assuming that I had supertoddler strength, let alone risking my safety on the bad old streets of London. But her expectations of me became my unquestioned expectations of myself, with the result that I have never queried my ability to meet a physical challenge.

All four of us children learned to swim and skate; there were ice shows and swimming galas. My brother was *victor ludorum* in athletics at his school and pursued his passion for sport by chucking up a safe career in engineering in his twenties to become a ski instructor. My two sisters became professional dancers. I wanted to dance too, but somehow that was not part of the plan. Diving was a good substitute. At ten I made probably one of the only important decisions of my life – I gave up swimming to concentrate on diving.

There followed idyllic years; diving every day, weekend courses, competitions all over the country, club nights, aquashows, thirty divers aged from five to fifty somersaulting off the high board to Wagner's 'The Ride of the Valkyries'; friends, dances, winning the Nationals, losing the Nationals, in-jokes, catch-phrases, thirteen of us in Rory's old Rover with the door tied on with string, tea and toast each night in the Italian caff after training, and on and on. Isn't nostalgia wonderful!

I was picked to dive internationally for the first time at age sixteen. It was a match between Great Britain and Germany held in Liverpool the same weekend as my O-Level Physics and Chemistry exams. At first it looked as if it would have to be a choice between schoolwork and diving. But, with great initiative, my Headmistress arranged for me to take the exams at Liverpool University. Whilst the rest of the team were down at the pool training, I took the exams, sitting in a vast, lofty, steeply raked lecture theatre with just the invigilator for company. This may sound like a sad story but it wasn't. I passed the exams and came second in the competition. That weekend marked the beginning of seven years of international competition, Commonwealth Games, European Championships and Olympics. I developed quite a taste for foreign travel.

It was the heyday of British diving and it

Right: *Liz diving for a bronze medal at the 1960 Olympic Games in Rome*

8

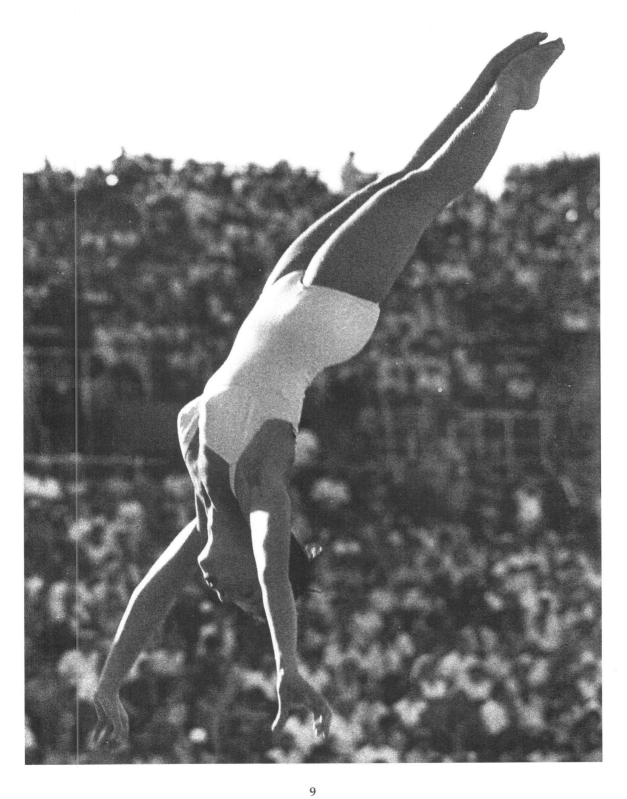

showed in the results. At the Olympic Games in Rome in 1960, Brian Phelps won a Bronze on the Highboard, the first British men's diving medal ever. I won a Bronze on the Spring-board, the first British medal in women's div-ing for forty years. Although Britain has had good divers since, in particular, Chris Snode who was double Commonwealth Champion in 1978 and 1982 and World Cup Champion in 1979, there have been no Olympic diving medals for Great Britain since 1960.

When, in 1964, I decided to stop diving, I had achieved almost everything I could have hoped for. I was at medical school and a dec-ision had to be made. It was time to hang up the 'cossie'. Faced with the dilemma of trying to fit in training when on 24-hour call to the obstetrics unit, delivering babies won hands down. The 'cossie' did get used occasionally. I swam for London University and was awarded a 'Purple' which is like an Oxbridge 'Blue' without the hype or the kudos.

My exercise regime was reduced to walking the hospital corridors – not to be sneezed at, but hardly comparable to an élite athlete's training programme.

From then till now I have not consistently followed an exercise regime, although the urge has certainly taken me from time to time – for instance, when the water in the pool is 80 degrees, the sun is shining in a cloudless sky and there is absolutely nothing else to do. Then I will swim laps endlessly. One of the problems about getting fit is that you have to do more and more exercise to maintain your fitness. You start by doing ten or twenty laps and feeling pleasantly tired afterwards; after a week that is no longer enough to produce this warm, contented glow and you have to in-crease the work. (I'll explain why in Chapter 8.)

There were occasional sustained bursts of energy, sometimes in the service of vanity or just after a birthday – very effective for focus-ing the mind. I enjoyed Lotte Berk's exercise classes on and off for years, mainly due to Lotte's continuous stream of saucy patter. It was a clever ploy to keep us distracted so that we hardly noticed the pain until attempting to climb the stairs after class when the knee wob-ble was fairly paralysing.

I even lived out my dancing fantasy by join-ing in at the back of Sophie's ballet class.

I look now at the dust gathering on the exer-cise bicycle in my bedroom and remember the times during the last twenty years when I have, yet again, started a 'new' exercise regime. On average, the enthusiasm lasted anything from two weeks to three months. I sold the idea to myself by saying that I could really sustain this exercise programme because it was so convenient and adaptable. I sounded like the salesman who had sold it to me, and yet, each time I set off on my bike ride to nowhere, I *knew* that the relentless tedium would eventually douse my already fragile en-thusiasm, leaving it as limp as an overcooked mange-tout.

What had happened to my will-power, to that single-minded self-discipline that élite athletes are supposed to have in abundance, so much so that you can almost see it popping out of every pore? Where was the drive and the tunnel vision? To distract my mind while pedalling, I listened to 'Gardener's Question Time' – although I didn't have a garden. Television provided some respite but the choice between cartoons and re-runs of 'I Love Lucy' did not exactly sustain my iron will. I even dug an old music stand out of the garage and set it up so that I could read a book, but the wind from the window, necessarily open to cool my sweating brow, kept making the page turn before I had finished reading it!

I was also a compulsive joiner of health clubs. I love all those black and chrome machines, steam rooms and peach-scented shampoo and body lotion. As I was pampered in pink towels amongst the potted plants, sipping peppermint tea, I felt just a tiny bit uneasy. Whilst I take exception to the alternative ethos of the cramped gym smelling of BO and sweaty socks, it seemed almost sinful to enjoy so much luxury in pursuit of fitness and health. But, of course, exercise has to be enjoyable and fun or people simply give up doing it. My discomfort, and the fact that these apparently healthy businesses had a habit of failing when I still had half a year of my subscription to run, meant I did not realize the full benefit of my investment. It seems that convenience and comfort were not enough. Vital ingredients were missing in my quest to find the perfect activity for me to stay fit and healthy. I lacked a goal – a target for which I

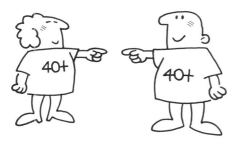

could train and which, with a bit of effort, I could achieve.

Then I ran into some triathletes – crazy people whose sport involves swimming, cycling and running for considerable distances, one after the other without a break. They were a close-knit bunch of loonies and I felt an immediate rapport! The sport of triathlon is still quite young and these splendid people evoked memories of the enthusiasm and commitment that I had experienced in my early days as a diver.

I thought there was only one kind of triathlon, the Ironman. Competitors in this event swim for 2½ miles in cold, unruly seas; then (still wet) jump on their bikes with only time to put on their shoes, and cycle for 112 miles; and follow this with a full marathon (26.2 mile) race. They had to be quite mad. The triathlon was not for me.

My new friends told me that there were much shorter triathlons and that the swimming often took place in swimming pools; that there were biathlons of cycling and running only; that there were mini-triathlons where the run was as short as two miles; that there were age-group competitions; and, finally, that anyone who started off with swimming as their strong sport (as I did) had a natural advantage. I was gently but surely being sucked into, and sold, the sport. More importantly, I was buying it hook, line and sinker!

Some weeks passed and the idea of doing triathlon simmered away somewhere in the back of my mind. The name and address of someone who organized triathlon training in my area magically appeared in the post, but the idea did not really come to the fore again until I met Andy for the first session of planning and organizing this book.

I discovered that he was already a seasoned triathlete while I had not even started on my first training outing. He enthused endlessly about the sport: how training for the three activities meant that boredom was not a problem; how a high degree of social contact contributed to his enjoyment of the sport, and how participants could be of any age from eighteen upwards within a broad spectrum of fitness and endurance.

Then it happened! I don't know quite how, but by some casual sleight of hand – I think it was to do with taking the dogs for a run – I found myself out on the recreation field running. I was being initiated very gently into a training programme for triathlon and to my great surprise I managed, with the gentlest of persuasion, to run and walk round that 600-metre field three times. By the time I had finished my chest screamed to stop, my head pounded with blood and my legs felt like balloons filled with heavy water.

'We'll enter you for the East Grinstead triathlon,' said Andy.

'I've never been to East Grinstead,' I panted.

'All the more reason!'

Three days later I was out on the rec. again with Sophie and the dogs. Sophie roared past me several times practising her sprinting. I plodded on and did my three revolutions, running, walking, running, and at the end of it I felt supremely smug. An old man walking his dog called out to me, 'Training for the marathon are you, or just trying to get a bit of the excess off?' Out of the mouths of babes

and old men. . . .

Two days later, I was in the pool with twenty other triathletes, pounding up and down, swimming length after length of freestyle; kick, pull and kick again. I couldn't believe that here I was doing the very thing that had so bored me at the age of ten that I had run away to diving at the first opportunity. Even more surprisingly, I was actually enjoying it. People were cheery and said things like, 'You seem to have done this kind of thing before.' The coach said I had a very good relaxed style and I felt childishly appreciative of this little bit of praise and encouragement. At 11 o'clock, I emerged into a dark, dank, drizzly night – and remembered those winters during my teens when I took four buses from Wembley to Isleworth in order to dive for forty-five minutes and then took four buses back. I got into my nice warm car and thought, 'East Grinstead, here I come!'

Andy's story

Although I was born in Liverpool, I went to a comprehensive school in Bristol, now closed down. I never trained or practised or specialized in any sport but took part in as many activities as there were opportunities. I even made it into the school orchestra, playing the cello, really badly. I played left back in the school Under-15 football team and was pretty average, although I did get a trial in the Bristol Public and Grammar School team. I ran in the school cross-country team in the winter and the athletics team in the summer.

My sporting love was canoeing. I wasn't very good at it. Pixie Wainwright, the wood-

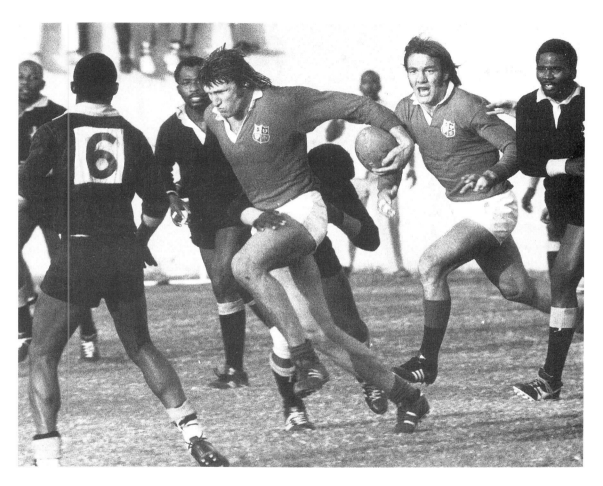

Andy in action for the British Lions in 1974

work master, helped a couple of us, in the lunch hour and after school (funded in my case by a paper round) build a marine ply-wood kayak each. I wasn't very good at wood-work either. I can still vividly remember my less than sturdy kayak on its maiden voyage, momentarily blocking the River Wye at Builth Wells. Filling up with water. Snapping in two. Me, slipping down the rapids crying, holding on to the paddle. We never found the canoe.

I took up rugby in my first year at university because I had grown too big and clumsy for soccer. In my final year, I started to run. Not far. Not fast. But I felt it was good for me, and I enjoyed it. From that time, I've done some form of exercise most days.

By the time I was twenty-eight I had won twenty-five England caps, played for the

Table I
Andy Ripley: training schedule (at 28 years old)

SUMMER	Morning/Lunchtime	Evening
Monday	rest	warm-up*: 4×200m rolling starts in 25, 24, 23, 22 secs 10 min recovery warm-down
Tuesday	free weights: bench press reps 6×6 @ 175lbs 4-mile lunchtime jog – 28 mins	warm-up: 300m, 500m, 300m, 500m in 40, 65, 40, 70 secs 10 min recovery warm-down
Wednesday	rest	warm-up: 100m-125m-150m pyramid near to maximum 5 min recovery warm-down
Thursday	free weights: bench press reps 6×6 @ 175lbs 4-mile lunchtime jog – 28 mins	warm-up: 10×100m strides and technique
Friday	rest**	rest**
Saturday	competition: usually 400m & 110m hurdles, high jump, one leg of 4×100m and 4×400m relay	
Sunday	long, easy jog 7 miles around Richmond Park	

WINTER	Morning/Lunchtime	Evening
Monday	hard (by my standards) run: 5 miles in 30 mins	rest
Tuesday	rest	stamina training at club
Wednesday	easy run: 4 miles in 28 mins	rest
Thursday	rest	stamina training and drills at club
Friday	rest**	rest**
Saturday	rugby match (afternoon)	rest
Sunday	long, easy jog (post-match condition permitting)	

* Summer warm-up routine: 4 very slow laps of track; 15 mins slow stretching; 5 laps walking with bends, stride straights; 1 lap walking; 5 mins stretching. Warm-down: 2 laps jogging.

** I've always enjoyed Fridays.

Summer training usually on tartan track in training group. Winter training in gym or at rugby (athletic) club ground.

British Lions, and won the TV 'Superstars' title. Table 1 shows a typical winter and summer training schedule. I was at my physical peak – playing my best rugby. However my best-ever athletics performance was failing to make the 1978 AAA 400-metres hurdles final by one place. The two sports, rugby and athletics, have a different approach to fitness which is essentially as follows.

Athletes usually train in kind weather, are highly tuned and sensitive to every sign and signal and, if the competition is important and they feel they won't do themselves justice, they will do anything not to compete. This is entirely understandable since winning and losing, or even doing well or badly, is measured in fractions of a second. I have known sensible guys looking for a time of, say, 10.5 in the 100 metres, doing 10.75 and, as a consequence, becoming suicidal. Athletes are individualistic, single-minded and dedicated. Their training consists of long periods of stretching and warming-up and very short periods at maximum or near to maximum effort. Training for athletes is on the margin, it's like making a 4H pencil even sharper. They achieve an intensity of effort in that short period of training unknown to most rugby players. They are also, by and large, a psychiatrist's dream – or nightmare.

If athletes live in the world of 4H then rugby players are definitely HB. A rugby player, who usually trains in the cold and wet, suffering from tonsilitis, a broken hand and a divorce, will always want to play. A dressing-room before a game is often like a casualty ward as players strap themselves up. I have not only known players with the most grue-some of injuries playing on, but also players to go on to the field in the full knowledge that they could hardly stand up, let alone walk. This attitude extends to training. Training is essentially stamina-based. It is not easier than athletics training, just different: a short warm-up, hanging around practising drills, interspersed with masses of low quality volume-repetition work. Surprisingly, rugby players are usually well adjusted.

At thirty-five, I enjoyed being the older player in the rugby and athletics teams long after my peers had given up. I carried on with the training schedule but, toward the end of my thirties, it became less important. In the summer my athletics training at the track ground to a halt and I ran less frequently and less hard around the village cricket field. I'd always wanted to be the best and, as my 40th birthday approached, I felt I could still make a contribution and the other players seemed to like me being there. Then, one day in 1989, I had a feeling that one or two players didn't need me around any more. I said nothing, maybe I was overly sensitive, but I decided to finish playing that season. I played my last game for Rosslyn Park against Cardiff on 23 April 1989, waved farewell a week or so later at the Middlesex Sevens and retired from rugby. I'd run the petrol right out of the tank. The game gave me so much, but the time was right. I hung up my boots, but not my trainers.

I missed the competition, the pre-match fear. Not the physical fear of being hurt, but the anticipation of losing or winning. Twenty-five years of biffing and carrying around 17 stone had also taken their toll on my knees. I had some X-rays taken. 'No real problem with your knees,' said the Expert. 'You're forty-three and your joints are getting tired, so don't do so much pounding on the streets.'

So I bought a bike, went swimming and started competing in short-course triathlons, in the 'good for his age' category. Being sociable I joined clubs, The East Grinstead Cycling Club, Triathlon Club and Weir Wood Sailing Club amongst others.

Rugby has given me up, my knees ache whenever I run, and Mother Nature is showing me no mercy. So why should I bother? Why not relax? After all that running round in circles don't I deserve to put my feet up and take it easy? But I still want to be active, to *live*, to compete.

Generously, Rosslyn Park asked me to be their president. Kingston Poly AC asked me to be a vice-president. But I don't want just to watch – I want to *do*. I have always exercised. Not because I'm afraid of heart disease – I need more motivation than the fear that I'll die one day. I enjoy exercise for its own sake. And I need to be competitive – not just against others but more importantly against myself.

I try to run three times a week, with the dog, not fast (7–8-minute miles), not far (3–5 miles). I do it when it's easy to fit it in. It's just part of my life. Wherever I am I usually carry some kit in my bag. I swim on Saturday mornings at the local leisure pool with the triathlon club, 8.00 till 9.00, and in the summer I do a bit more. I join the guys sometimes for an open-water swim, if I'm feeling brave.

I cycle from March till October, perhaps an early Sunday morning ride across Ashdown Forest (30 miles) before the cars wake up and 10-mile time trials on Wednesday evenings.

I compete in about five triathlons a year, do a few fun runs and anything else that seems a good idea.

I no longer have a need to run as fast as I can over 400 metres, or charge at big men in different coloured shirts, but at forty-three I do need to look after myself by taking regular, gentle exercise. *And so do you.*

Throughout my life I've set myself short-term goals which are testing but attainable. You can set targets for any goal you want to achieve – be it losing weight, making money, passing an exam, painting the house, or running a marathon. The principles are the same:

✷ Set yourself a testing but attainable target, to be achieved by a specific date

✷ Plan how you're going to get there

✷ Write it down and commit yourself to it

✷ Have the discipline to do it

✷ Record what you have done

The target I set myself was to check out five new exercise activities suitable for a man of Forty-something

✷ sailing

✷ swimming

✷ cycling

✷ golf

✷ the Health Club

In chapter 10 you'll find out how I got on.

I also decided to watch my eating habits. Although I still weigh the same as I did when I gave up rugby, I'm aware that I've lost muscle. I've never worried about my body shape, but now with an exercise programme that takes into account I'm a forty-three-year-old man, it would be a smart move to lose some weight before it becomes a problem. Up till now, I've always eaten as much as I like, whenever I wanted, and I've never dieted. I feel the reason I haven't put on weight is that I drink alcohol infrequently and I exercise every day. I think I have a reasonably balanced diet, but I eat meat, have sugar in my coffee, eat white bread and like butter and cream. On a Saturday morning I really enjoy a heart-stopping breakfast of fried eggs, five rashers of bacon, loads of toast and fried bread. I love

chocolate and find it quite easy to polish off a box of Maltesers, two Crunchies and a Turkish Delight in one session. But if I do want to lose weight and improve my health, now is the time to think about eating less and eating better.

Incidentally, I've never smoked. I never liked it. When I was fourteen my elder brother Mike, who wanted to play football for England, found two Wills Weights that Johnny Philips had stolen from his grandmother, in my drawer. I liked my brother, he told me it was dumb to smoke. He was right then and he's still right now.

Andy, the family man

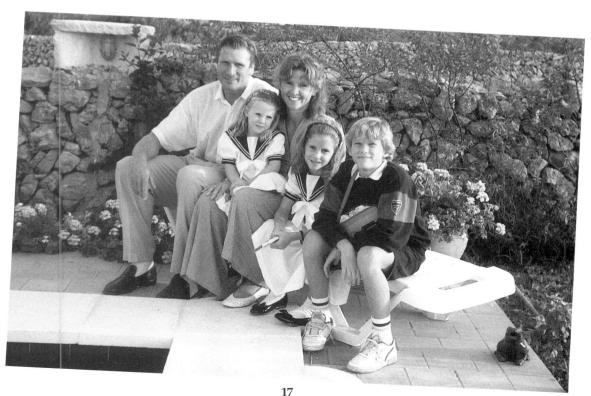

THREE

Ageing – What you are up against

Hippocrates said 2400 years ago:

Speaking generally, all parts of the body which have a function, if used in moderation and exercised in labours to which each is accustomed, become thereby healthy and well developed, and age slowly; but if un-used and left idle they become liable to disease, defective in growth, and age quickly.

Withington, E.T. (trans): Hippocrates, *New York, Putnam Publishing Group, 1927 (Volume 3)*

No one wants to get old. Some people, it's true, may approach the business of ageing with grace and fortitude, philosophically acknowledging its inevitability and even curiously anticipating the calm and peace that physical and mental slowing may bring. But such composed acquiescence is rare.

It is more common to find people facing the prospect of getting older (if indeed they face it at all) with reluctance and distaste. Some manage to deny it is happening, sometimes with quite comic results. Others ignore it as much as possible, conveniently forgetting their own birthdays and the dates of various life milestones.

Ageing is a condition that creeps up on you – a decline so gradual that you hardly know it is happening. What is the odd, grey hair or a few laughter lines? Surely, these are signs of maturity, not age? It takes a look of disbelief on the face of a 'long-time-no-see' friend to drive home the awful truth. One gets a sneaky feeling that the surprised greeting 'I didn't recognize you!', really means 'You look so old!'. The worst of it is that you may still *feel* twenty-five and, at times, act a lot younger even than that.

If your heart is sinking, fear not – you are not alone. The quest for eternal youth and long life has always been a human obsession. Until fairly recently, mystical views held sway, characterized in medieval times by the search for an elixir or fifth essence (*quinta essentia*) as a 'cure' for ageing. Before ageing became the subject of scientific study, there were a number of myths about it.

One was that the human body contained a certain amount of essential spirit or life which was gradually depleted with age, resulting eventually in disease and death. From this image came the idea of the ageing body being like a candle gradually spluttering out, or a leaf withering, or a well gradually emptying. People believed that the human body had a fixed quantity of life and that when this amount of life had run its course, as at the end of the day, the shadows would lengthen, the hour glass empty, the sun set and the road end.

Persistent interest in longevity and rejuvenation has stimulated the recently developed sciences of molecular biology and neuroendocrinology, as well as those of clinical medicine and physiology, to invest considerable resources in attempting to unravel the mystery of the ageing process.

We begin to age from the moment of conception and continue until we die. Change and development are occurring in the body all the time; for example, the onset of puberty signals in both sexes the start of reproductive life, whilst the menopause identifies its end in women. These are normal developmental milestones although the age at which they occur varies considerably from individual to individual. Nevertheless, these major physical and physiological changes are easily identifiable.

Other changes associated with ageing are much more subtle; it is difficult to trace their beginning because the tiny incremental changes go unnoticed from one day to the next. The gums gradually recede to give the 'long in the tooth' look, the teeth become yellow, 'age spots' appear on sagging, wrinkling skin; the body gets shorter and broader as if a huge hammer has been tap, tap, tapping away on the top of the head – a person can shrink by as much as one-and-a-half inches between thirty and seventy years of age. The spine curves and 'a dowager's hump' may appear. The abdomen swells as extra fat is stored around the gut. The nose and ears can grow bigger and a forest of hair appear in their orifices. Blue-black veins may bulge out tortuously from swollen legs. Get the picture?

As well as these unwelcome changes in appearance there is the equally, if not more, distressing loss of function. For most people, getting older means being able to *do* less and finding it harder to complete tasks which were once done without effort. Awareness dawns, often painfully, of the limitations of the body; muscle strength, flexibility and endurance can no longer be taken for granted; joints creak and click, muscles waste and weaken; running for a bus, walking up a hill carrying a load of shopping, or leaning into a strong head wind, become too much effort – the heart pounds, breathing is laboured and the muscles ache with fatigue.

Sexual activity usually wanes even if interest is sustained. Hearing often deteriorates

> **' It's a sign of age if you feel like the day after the night before and you haven't been anywhere. '**

and memory becomes unreliable. Opening the early morning post may require the tiresome donning of the little gold-rimmed half specs. A decline in vision is almost universal and indicates without doubt that middle age has well and truly arrived. As the saying goes, 'You are getting old when the gleam in your eyes is from the sun reflecting off your bifocals.' In other words, most people expect that with age their looks will gradually change for the worse and their activities will gradually and inexorably be curtailed.

Hand-in-hand with the changes in the body that begin to occur from thirty–forty years of age, comes the increased risk of chronic disease. In more developed countries a greater number of people are living to a ripe old age today than at the turn of the century, owing to the drastically reduced death toll from infectious diseases with the discovery of antibiotics and vaccines. But another kind of epidemic has replaced those due to micro-organisms. This epidemic consists of a cluster of conditions known as the chronic diseases of civilization – heart disease, cancer, diabetes, hypertension, obesity, strokes, lung diseases, osteoporosis (brittle bones) and arthritis. Those at risk are the middle-aged, 'healthy' individuals of the Western world.

Why do we age?

When Jesus Christ died, aged thirty-three, he had attained the average life-span for that era. In 1900, the average age of death in the UK was fifty; today it is about seventy for men and seventy-five for women. All through history, there have been those who have survived longer than expected (Moses, for instance, is believed to have lived to 120). The difference today is that more people than ever before are living to a greater age because fewer people die prematurely from disease and trauma. However, the *maximum* life-span has not altered. According to scientific records, no human being has managed to survive beyond 120 years.

Why do people die? It seems that, like every other living creature, humans are programmed for extinction with the human age limit genetically determined. A fruitfly lives a few hours whilst a Galapagos tortoise may live for well over 100 years. But, whatever the lifespan, it is all in the genes of a particular species. What happens to cause the eventual demise?

1. *The theory of 'intrinsic limitation'* suggests that cells are only capable of a limited number of divisions before they die. There may be a gene that causes self-destruction of the cell or a 'killer hormone' that finally annihilates it.

2. *The 'wear and tear' theory* suggests that, with advancing age, damage due to infection and disease destroys the cells and causes pathological changes because the immune system that normally defends the body by producing antibodies is faulty.

3. *The error theory* proposes that a mistake is made in the synthesis of protein in the cell due to 'wrong' information from the DNA in the genes. DNA (deoxyribonucleic acid) and RNA (ribonucleic acid) are the bearers or messengers of coded information that directs the cell to behave in a particular way – for instance, as a liver cell or a muscle cell, etc. If the DNA/RNA bears a wrong code, the cell behaves differently from normal, just as a ship set on the wrong course will end up at a wrong destination. If enough cells in a particular organ or tissue get the wrong message, that organ will not function properly. Eventually, like a row of dominoes falling over, the whole organism will fail to thrive.

Errors arise from irradiation damage to DNA, free radicals breaking up the DNA (see page 25), the effects of drugs, certain dietary components like nitrosamines, or toxic chemicals that produce solid waste products, such as pigments, that act like 'clinkers' in a furnace, getting in the way of normal function.

When cells degenerate and die for whatever reason the organs and systems of the body run down and become inefficient. When critical elements of any system break down, the entire system will eventually stop functioning – like broken traffic lights at a busy intersection. In the face of attack from environmental stresses and insults like irradiation, drugs, pollution, poor nutrition, tobacco smoke and other carcinogens (i.e. entities that trigger the cancer process in cells), heat and cold, bacteria and other infections, the body, like a warrior without his weapons, finally succumbs.

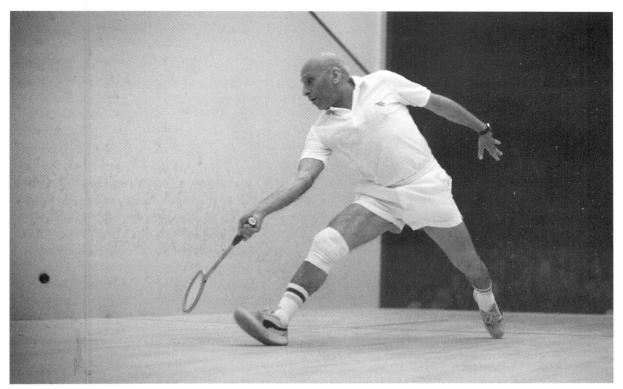

Hashim Khan played top-class squash until he was well over forty – and also taught Liz to play

In health, there is a natural tendency for the body to stabilize its 'internal environment', a process referred to as *homeostasis*. For example, when the body temperature tends to rise in extreme heat or during endurance exercise, mechanisms come into play to reduce it to normal, such as sweating and increased flow of blood to the skin, making it turn red. Being able to meet the broadest spectrum of possible challenges – physical, mental and emotional – is the key to health and well-being.

Up to the age of forty, the majority of us seem to assume with a degree of unquestioning arrogance that we can defy any thrusts of fortune that gratuitously come our way, deftly parrying and volleying with impudent assurance, rarely doubting our might or main.

Even when things go badly wrong and we founder, feeling wretched and defeated, there is an assumption that sooner or later a fair wind will blow and all will be well again. Forty is something of a watershed; it is the time when people take out life insurance. Although not quite 'over the hill', it is as if we have reached the top and can see down the other side. Confidence gained through four decades of living and loving is counterbalanced by concern for a fearful future.

As we get older, the homeostatic mechanisms that enable the body to meet and overcome the profusion of challenges that crowd our daily lives become sluggish and inefficient. Exposure to any variation from the norm, whether it is heat, cold, altitude, diet, infection or disease, is a stress to the body. With age, the reserves that normally deal with these stresses become depleted. An individual has less ability to respond to sudden or unexpected demands for strength, speed and quick reaction. Eventually, even quite ordinary activities may become too much, at which point a person can become disabled and dependent.

Cause for optimism

This demise with age may be considered 'normal' but, fortunately, it is not necessarily natural. The average age of the population is increasing. In 1990, people over forty numbered 24.7 million in the UK, which is 43% of the total population. By the year 2000, the over-forties will count for nearly 46% of the total. No longer 'old' at sixty or sixty-five, people can look forward to fifteen or twenty years of 'active' retirement if they can remain healthy and hardy.

Not everyone ages at the same rate. Some people weather well whilst others look and grow old before their time. The biological clock of ageing is not synchronized with the passing of years. Those people who retain their youthful vigour seem to have managed to slow the biological clock down relative to their actual chronological age. Why do some people stay younger longer? Genetics undoubtedly play an important part – youthfulness does seem to run in families. But they do not tell the whole story.

There is evidence of certain isolated communities in Kashmir, Georgia, Ecuador and Okinawa where there are high proportions of centenarians living vigorous and active lives. Studies have shown that all these peoples have two things in common: (1) a diet which is rich in unrefined wholefoods like cereals and rice and is significantly lower in calories and fat than that of the Western world in general, and (2) a physically active lifestyle throughout their lives.

A similarly long-lived group is the non-smoking, non-drinking Seventh Day Adventists, one in eight of whom live to be over ninety. They too are prone to carry on moderate to heavy physical activity until well into their eighties and nineties.

The evidence from these populations suggests that vitality and long life are related to lifestyle, especially diet and physical activity. Ways of slowing down the ageing process are examined later in this chapter.

What happens as we age?

The questions to which we all want to know the answers are: (1) What happens to the body and its functions after forty? (2) What can we do to slow down, prevent or even reverse the effects of ageing? These are the questions which I will attempt to answer here.

The brain is at its heaviest in the early twenties (approximately 1.4 kg). Thereafter it undergoes a slow decline, the loss of weight reaching 7%, or about 100g, by age eighty. Brain cells, like muscle cells, cannot regenerate and throughout life they are lost at an estimated rate of 50,000 per day out of a total of 10 billion. Alarming as these figures may appear at first, in fact only about 3% of total nerve cells are lost in a lifetime. Men's brains deteriorate at a faster rate than those of women, in particular those parts of the brain responsible for the higher functions unique to humans – logical reasoning, language, calculating, conceptualizing and emotions; no one knows why, but the sex hormones are thought to be involved and, the experts say, may explain why old men tend to be grumpier than old women!

Bone becomes thinner in both sexes as it loses calcium after about thirty-five years of age; this loss accelerates in women after the menopause as oestrogen levels fall, causing osteoporosis (brittle bones) which predisposes to fractures.

Whilst bone-loss appears to be a normal part of the ageing process, a sedentary lifestyle plays an important contributing role.* Even young people confined to bed for long periods due to illness suffer loss of bone. So do astronauts in space who are without the pull of gravity. Bones need the stimulation of the pull of tendons and contracting muscles, plus the force of gravity, to maintain their strength and thickness.

Joints become less flexible as the fibrous tissue surrounding them increases and becomes more dense; movement is limited as a result – it is more difficult to scratch your back as you get older.

Muscle strength and size are greatest between twenty and thirty years of age. Thereafter, speed and power gradually diminish as muscles become smaller and weaker due to a reduction in the number and size of muscle fibres. Chronic low-back problems, which are among the commonest reasons that adults consult a doctor, occur when those 'pillars of strength' – the back and abdominal muscles that support the spine – become wasted and weak.

*Women endurance athletes and ballet dancers who stop menstruating due to abnormally low oestrogen levels are also prone to premature bone-loss similar to that seen in post-menopausal women.

Similar painful problems are common in the shoulder, hip and knee, when weak muscles combine with stiff joints, the latter due to loss of elasticity and increased rigidity of connective tissue in the tendons and ligaments around the joint. Lack of regular physical exercise results in loss of strength, speed, power and agility. Muscles grow stronger and joints more flexible if they are used. Exercise programmes that focus on muscle strengthening and flexibility (see pages 99-106) have produced excellent results in people with muscle and joint conditions.

Skin loses its elasticity and becomes increasingly rigid in its deeper layers, resulting in wrinkles, lines and a coarse texture. In addition, skin cells, that are like plump plums

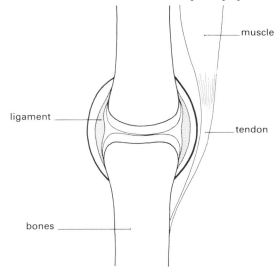

Figure 1 Reduction of muscle fibre combined with loss of elasticity in the tendons and ligaments causes stiff and painful knees

when young, lose much of their water and become like pitted prunes, giving ageing skin its characteristic dry, loose, cracked appearance. The pigment-producing cells become less active, leaving the skin pale and bloomless, and the hair grey.

Lungs lose their elasticity and the chest deepens from front to back as the ribs fail to be pulled in by the lungs' elastic recoil, giving the appearance of a puffed-up pigeon. Residual, stale air is left in the lungs with each breath, so breathing is inefficient and lung infections and bronchitis are prevalent.

Lean body mass (LBM), otherwise known as fat-free tissue, diminishes from age forty onwards, principally due to loss of bone, wasting of muscles and a decrease in the size of virtually all organs, especially the liver and kidneys. Since the body is housing a smaller engine, the energy needed to keep it going is less and food requirements decrease. But food intake generally does not change or may even increase; the result is that the excess food/ energy is stored as fat. *Too much food and too little exercise are the principal causes of overweight in middle age.*

In countries where food is short, people do not get fatter as they get older. Also, studies of athletes taking part in Veterans' and Masters' competitions have shown them to be no fatter in their sixties, seventies or eighties than active young people. Overweight is not a *necessary* accompaniment of ageing, but the almost ubiquitous appearance of the middle-age spread has important associations with the onset of chronic disease, in particular,

heart disease, high blood pressure, diabetes and certain cancers.

Blood vessels become increasingly rigid and inflexible; the blood pressure tends to rise and damage to the lining of the vessels occurs. Like the banks of a river that are eroded by the current, the walls of blood vessels are susceptible to damage by the flow of blood, especially at the bends in the arteries. These 'wounds' cause an inflammatory response and scar tissue forms which attracts deposits of fatty plaques of cholesterol in the walls – a condition that is exaggerated in people with high blood cholesterol levels. As a result of these accumulations of fat, the vessels become narrower – a condition known as atherosclerosis – and the blood flow is reduced so that less oxygen reaches the tissues. In addition, blood clots may form that can plug a small vessel. If this happens in a coronary artery supplying heart muscle, a portion of the muscle dies from lack of oxygen. In other words, the individual suffers from a *heart attack*.

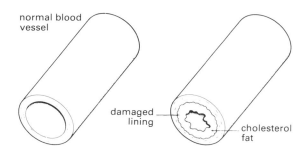

Figure 2 What happens to blood vessels with age and cholesterol

If the blockage is incomplete, but some part of the heart muscle is still deprived of oxygen, severe pains in the chest are felt, known as *angina*; this pain is most frequently felt during exertion when the oxygen demands on the heart are greatest. In addition to increasing the risk of a heart attack, the change in the blood vessels may cause a stroke and predispose towards premature death. (See also pages 52-54 High-fat Diet.)

The catalogue of age-related changes listed above, that gradually happens in the body after forty, falls broadly into two categories:

1. Rigidity, inelasticity and inflexibility of tissues, e.g. skin, tendons, fibrous joint capsules, lungs and blood vessels.

2. Loss of tissue with accompanying decline in function accelerated by lack of use, e.g. in muscles, bones and heart.

Rigidity of tissues with age happens as bundles of collagen and elastin that form the support system in organs and tissues all over the body literally become 'tied' together. Collagen and elastin are part of an all-pervasive supporting network called connective tissue that not only 'connects' the body's structures, one with another, but also exists between the cells of skin, muscles, tendons, bone, cartilage, blood vessels and all the structural supports that give the body its shape and substance, as well as in organs like the liver, kidneys, stomach, gut, glands, etc.

In a young person, collagen fibres are soft and flexible, whilst elastin has the ability to

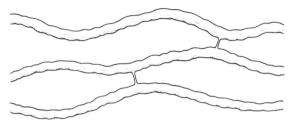

collagen fibres in youthful connective tissue – flexible and supple with only a few cross-linkages

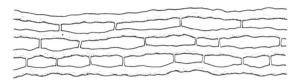

collagen fibres in forty-plus connective tissue – rigid and inelastic due to increased cross-linkages between the fibres

Figure 3   Tissues become more rigid with age as cross-linkages form

stretch and recoil. With age, collagen thickens and becomes dense and rigid as **cross-linkages** form that bind the bundles tightly together; elastin loses its elasticity and becomes fatigued like the over-stretched elastic in old underwear.

The formation of cross-linkages contributes more than anything else to the ageing process in tissue and is due to the action of **free radicals**.

Free radicals are by-products of the use in human and animal cells of oxygen in the combustion of food to produce energy for life. Although the use of oxygen to produce life energy in evolutionary terms conveys a significant advantage over earlier forms of life that could not support the presence of oxygen, the downside is the production of these

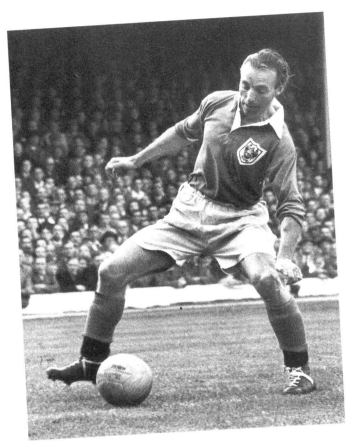

Stanley Matthews played in the First Division when he was fifty

highly reactive, unstable atoms that are literally set free from the molecules to which they belong when they meet oxygen. Normally, free radicals remain within the cell, but they may escape under the detrimental influence of pollutants in the atmosphere, ultra-violet irradiation or certain dietary substances. Then, true to their name, they are free to wander wherever the fancy takes them, their aim being to join up with other molecules. In doing so, they interrupt the functions of cells, damaging DNA and causing disruption of coded genetic information.

In connective tissue, free radicals react with protein in the cells or tissues to produce **cross-links**, both within and between the molecules. As a result, tissues which were soft and flexible like the skin of a baby's bottom become hard and rigid. It is as if molecules that used to be able to move easily around each other become stuck together in rigid chains, and the bundles of collagen and elastin in skin, muscles and ligaments, that used to be as pliable as young bamboo, become stiff and unyielding like the trunk of an old tree.

The destruction free radicals can cause in cells, distorting the information contained in the genes and other structures and wreaking havoc in the systems of the body, contributes to the development of the chronic degenerative conditions related to ageing – principally heart disease and cancer.

The body is not totally at the mercy of these molecular mad-caps. Free radicals can be disarmed of their potentially damaging effects by **antioxidants**, substances that occur naturally in all cells. Antioxidants can mop up the radicals before the genetic material is harmed.

Fortunately, in addition to naturally occurring antioxidants, supportive back-up can be provided by including in the diet foods rich in antioxidants – vitamins A, E and C, and beta-carotene and selenium. Dark green, leafy vegetables like cabbage, broccoli and watercress, as well as yellow vegetables and fruit like carrots, mango, apricot and citrus fruits, have an abundance of these vitamins and trace elements.

Besides slowing down the ageing process by neutralizing damaging free radicals, diets high in these fruits and vegetables are associated with a reduced risk of cancer and heart disease. A study found that Scottish men with angina had lower blood levels of vitamins A, C and E than those who did not have heart disease. In Mediterranean countries, where the diet contains a large proportion of fruit and vegetables, the populations have a significantly reduced risk of cancer and heart disease, and this is attributed to the antioxidant properties of these foods. (See also pages 58-60.)

Loss of tissue – bone, muscle, lean body mass – with ageing is no more than can be expected, since the natural behaviour pattern for all animals, humans included, is to become less and less active as they get older. Unfortunately, the less active people are, the more their physical capabilities deteriorate.

The 'normal' decline in stamina (measured as maximum oxygen uptake – VO_2 max) from 20–60 years is 10% per decade with women deteriorating at a slower rate than men. This decline in aerobic capacity goes hand-in-hand with less physical activity. Active people, however, can sustain their stamina levels for longer than those who are sedentary and fitness training from 40–60 years can alleviate this decline. The bonus of fitness training is that normal activities, like running for a bus or walking up stairs, are less of an effort. Reserves of energy are greater. Work can be done with more ease and comfort. Both heart rate and blood pressure are lower and heart muscle needs less oxygen for a given exercise effort, which is a particular benefit for a person over forty who may have a degree of narrowing of the coronary arteries.

The Good News is that many people can regain a great deal of what they may have lost in strength, agility and stamina if they pursue a regular exercise programme. Inevitable as ageing may be, many of the effects can be delayed with a regular fitness and strengthening programme. In fact, some aspects of the ageing process can even be reversed!

Stemming the tide

Vigorous fitness training in one's youth offers no benefit in later years if exercise training was stopped early on. The greatest runner in the world at twenty-five years of age could not sustain the stamina level of an élite athlete without continuing training. Equally, an individual following a regular exercise programme for the first time in middle age can receive all the benefits so long as he or she continues with it on a regular basis.

Weight-bearing exercise (e.g. running, jogging, dancing) is particularly beneficial for women, both pre- and post-menopausally, because not only can bone-loss be prevented but bone that has become thin can be rebuilt and strengthened. Weight-training exercise with free weights or machines can dramatically strengthen weak and wasted muscles even in ninety-year-olds. Physical exercise also enhances collagen metabolism, resulting in stronger tendons and ligaments which suggests that the characteristic loss of elasticity and increased rigidity in muscles and tendons with age are reversible with physical training.

These are examples of how some aspects of the ageing process can be *reversed* with physical exercise. Unfortunately, in this country it is often the case that on reaching a certain age – say fifty – individuals bend to what society regards as appropriate behaviour for their age and significantly reduce their physical activity. The general attitude as we get older is 'Don't exert yourself unless you absolutely have to.' Even hitherto active people tend to 'retire gracefully'; for instance, singles tennis is replaced with doubles, because less is expected of a person in doubles tennis.

A vicious circle begins in which less and less regular exercise is taken and, as a result, the ability to perform physical exercise diminishes. It seems that this gradually diminishing physical capacity is due to ageing when, in fact, it is associated with a progressively more sedentary lifestyle.

Clearly, lifestyle habits have a profound effect on the 'usual' pattern of ageing. In particular, it becomes increasingly clear that a lack of physical exercise undoubtedly contributes to a gradual deterioration in the whole body.

Nature's helpers

Besides a healthy diet and regular exercise, what other factors inhibit ageing?

The thymus gland weighs about half a pound at birth, begins to atrophy at puberty and is just a tiny collection of cells at sixty years of age. It secretes a hormone called thymosin, the purpose of which, until recently, was not

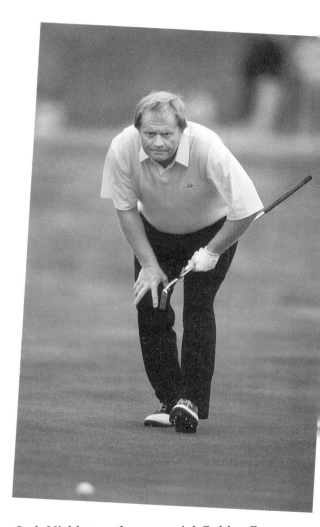

Jack Nicklaus – the perennial Golden Bear

known. Thymosin plays a critical role in the body's stress response; deterioration of the thymus with age produces deterioration of the brain and the whole body. The time is foreseen when thymosin may be taken to delay or arrest the effects of ageing.

The adrenal glands secrete a steroid, DHEA (dihydroepiandrosterone), which protects the thymus, thus maintaining high levels of thymosin. In the future, it is believed that synthetically produced high potency DHEA may be available which could make a sixty-year-old person appear twenty years younger.

Repair enzymes are produced by genes in cells when DNA is damaged and needs urgent assistance to maintain its integrity. Without this help, cells with damaged DNA degenerate and die. It is anticipated that, eventually, biologists will be able to manufacture repair enzymes which could then be taken like a food supplement to help cells stay healthy and young.

If you don't use it, you will certainly lose it!

The Methuselah gene is the name given to a gene that appears to offer the prospect of a long life. It is named after the biblical patriarch who is supposed to have lived for 900 years. It is believed to produce very high levels of high-density lipoprotein (HDL) cholesterol – five times the normal levels. HDL is the 'good' form of cholesterol that protects against heart disease by preventing clogging of the arteries and is, therefore, believed to promote longevity. It is conceivable that in the future, with gene therapy, the benefit of this 'long-life' gene could become widely available.

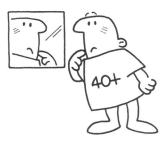

Hormone replacement therapy is increasingly commonplace for women, to ameliorate the symptoms of the menopause and, particularly, to prevent bone-loss and osteoporosis. Recently, male HRT has been in the news, somewhat controversially. Pioneer work in Denmark has shown that testosterone deficiency in middle-aged men may be associated with premature ageing of the heart and circulation. Testosterone replacement is believed by some to counteract the effects of the male 'viropause' and to revive feelings of vigour and vitality in men who feel 'over the hill'.

Human growth hormone (HGH), secreted by the pituitary gland, tends to decline after about age thirty and the decrease contributes to the increase in fatty tissue and decrease in muscle mass and bone density that occurs with ageing. A recent study showed that these changes could be reversed in men over sixty who were given HGH for six months. This work suggests that the administration of HGH to ageing people may have the potential for reversing some of the undesirable effects of the ageing process.

Nature's killers

In childhood and up to the age of thirty or so, survival depends for the most part on avoiding fatal accidents. For the over-forties, surviving to a vigorous old age may mean avoiding the killer diseases of our industrialized world that can strike a person down in their prime – in particular, heart disease. This book is about staying healthy and fit in the second half of life; to achieve this goal, a critical question is what to do in order to reduce the risk of heart disease.

Coronary Heart Disease (CHD) is the biggest single cause of premature death in Great Britain for both men and women. It accounts for nearly 150,000 deaths per year in total – about 30% of all male deaths and 23% of all female deaths. In world rankings, Northern Ireland has the highest death rate from CHD with Scotland a close second. England and Wales are not far behind in sixth place after Czechoslovakia, Finland and Eire; the death rates in this country are still six times higher than in Japan which has the lowest incidence in the world, followed closely by Italy and France.

It is unlikely that this remarkable variation is due to some intrinsic genetic or inherited difference between the people of Japan and those in the UK and other countries high up in the world rankings. Unlike infectious diseases such as tuberculosis, coronary heart disease does not have a single cause. Rather, it is a condition associated with a number of risk factors. Personal characteristics, such as genetic make-up, sex, age and race, may act as risk factors, but obviously these cannot be changed.

There are other CHD risk factors, however, influenced by a person's lifestyle, that *are* within the control of the individual:

* cigarette smoking

* obesity

* raised blood cholesterol

* raised blood pressure

* lack of physical exercise

* diabetes (of mature onset)

* alcohol

* stress

When more than one risk factor occurs together, the risk of a heart attack is considerably increased. If you are a cigarette smoker with high blood pressure and raised blood cholesterol, your risk of dying from CHD increases eight-fold.

So let's now examine in more detail the lifestyle habits that affect coronary heart disease (see Table 2, page 33):

CIGARETTE SMOKING

The substantial reduction in deaths due to CHD in recent years has been largely attributed to a decline in cigarette smoking. Between 1972 and 1986, the numbers of men

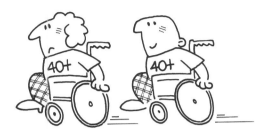

smoking in this country fell from 52% to 35% and the numbers of women fell from 41% to 31%. During the same period, there was a 39% reduction in CHD deaths in men aged 35–44, whilst the reduction among women of the same age was 40%.

WEIGHT CONTROL

Overweight is associated with raised blood pressure, raised blood cholesterol, diabetes and lack of physical exercise. Ideally, weight-loss can be achieved with a reducing diet combined with increased physical exercise. Both blood pressure and blood cholesterol are lowered by these measures and the risk of CHD is lessened.

NUTRITION

Diets high in fat, particularly saturated (animal) fat, are associated with high blood cholesterol levels. Cutting down on fatty foods and including more fibre-rich food in the diet, tends to lower blood cholesterol levels.

These changes will also help with weight-loss which, in turn, will have a beneficial effect if blood pressure is raised. Avoiding salt, both on and in food, also contributes to lowering a raised blood pressure.

Diets rich in vitamins E and C (wholegrain cereals, fruit, vegetables and vegetable oils) decrease the risk of CHD.

PHYSICAL ACTIVITY

A slothful, sedentary lifestyle often goes hand-in-hand with obesity which, in turn, can predispose to the kind of diabetes that develops in middle life. Physical activity, on the other hand, can reduce obesity, lower blood cholesterol and blood pressure. It also benefits diabetics, who are twice as likely to die of a heart attack as non-diabetics, by increasing insulin sensitivity.

Most importantly, evidence supports the view that physical activity operates independently of its effect on obesity, blood pressure and blood cholesterol, and has a direct effect on reducing the risk of heart disease by increasing blood flow to the heart muscle and improving its function.

ALCOHOL

Alcohol has a high calorie content (7 Kcal per gram). People who are heavy drinkers (56 units – see page 63 for definition of a unit – or more per week) are often overweight and have high blood pressure. Consuming less alcohol will help with weight-loss and will contribute to lowering blood pressure. (For other effects of alcohol, see Chapter 5, pages 61-63.)

STRESS

Most people believe that stress in everyday life, producing anxiety and often depression, has a strong link with the development of heart disease. The American cardiologists, Dr Meyer Friedman and Dr Ray Rosenman, legitimized this popular belief when they showed that more than 90% of the one in five American men who suffered a heart attack before the age of sixty showed a behaviour pattern that they labelled as 'Type A'. The Type A pattern is characterized by aggressiveness and competitiveness, a sense of urgency ('hurry sickness'), impatience and being in a chronic struggle to achieve more and more in less and less time. Type As seem to create stress at every turn, causing large amounts of stress hormones to course around their bodies, a condition to which they may well be addicted. (See pages 83-86.)

The result is an increased blood cholesterol level, and an increased blood pressure. Since these highly stressed individuals are likely to be cigarette smokers, probably take little or no exercise (they hardly have time) and may well be overweight, they 'take the biscuit' as far as being at risk of having a heart attack is concerned. (See also pages 39-40.)

Another study has shown a different kind of stress related to CHD. Immigrants from the Indian sub-continent have a mortality rate from heart disease that is 25% higher than the general population in this country. The difference is thought to be due not to diet, high blood pressure or cigarette smoking, but rather to the stress of migration.

You can do something about reducing stress in your life. Relaxation classes that included breathing exercises, meditation and stress management, held over a period of two months, had a significant lowering effect on raised blood pressure in a group at risk from heart disease, with the therapeutic effect persisting four years later. (See also pages 91-94.)

Public awareness during the last twenty years of the risk factors involved in heart disease in the UK has led to an overall drop in mortality of 21% in men and 15% in women. But, we have lagged considerably behind the USA and Australia where the decline in mortality from CHD is three times greater than here. In those countries, large numbers of the populations have been quicker to take up the challenge to change their behaviour by giving up cigarette smoking, eating low-fat diets and being more physically active, all of which are major factors in preventing heart disease (see Table 2).

Cancer is the commonest cause of premature death in women before they reach the menopause; until that age they are protected from heart disease by their hormones. But, in contrast to heart disease in which, as we have seen above, a change of lifestyle can have a protective effect, preventative measures in cancer are not as established. Nevertheless, a relationship has been suggested between cancer of the breast, a condition from which one in twelve women in this country suffer at some time in their lives, and a high-fat diet. In addition, the risk of colon cancer, which is related to ageing, is lowered by increased levels of physical activity because the time spent by food passing through the intestines is less,

Table 2 Lifestyle factors affecting heart disease

RISK FACTOR	LIFESTYLE HABITS					
	Not Smoking	Weight Control	Good Nutrition	Increased Physical Activity	Reduced Alcohol Intake	Stress Management
Cigarette Smoking	▨					
Raised Blood Pressure	▨	▨	▨	▨	▨	▨
Raised Cholesterol		▨	▨	▨		▨
Obesity		▨	▨	▨		
Lack of Exercise				▨		▨
Diabetes		▨	▨	▨		▨
Stress				▨		▨
Alcohol		▨	▨		▨	

▨ Positive effect of lifestyle habits on CHD Risk Factors

and so carcinogenic substances in the waste products spend less time in contact with the gut wall.

Summary

In a sense, ageing is inevitable while we live in a world of four dimensions. Until astronauts turn our traditional concept of 'absolute' time upside down by returning from prolonged space travel younger than when they left this planet, we are destined to chug along from birth to death becoming progressively more worn and torn, wrinkled and rigid, as the far side of the hill is reached. But, as we have seen, we can slow down and even reverse the ravaging effects of passing time by engaging in a lifestyle that focuses on good nutrition and regular physical activity plus avoidance of irradiation (sun or other), exposure to toxic chemicals and harmful substances in food. When these anti-ageing measures are combined with not smoking, weight control, moderate alcohol intake and stress management, the chances of living a long healthy life by avoiding disease and premature death are significantly increased.

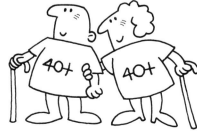

FOUR

Smoking or Non-Smoking

In recent years, cigarette smoking has received a pretty bad press, as awareness of the associated dangers to health have seeped into public consciousness. Tobacco advertising in newspapers, magazines, cinemas, on billboards and on the outside of shops selling tobacco products will soon be banned. But, because of the loophole allowing sponsorship of sport, tobacco advertising on television has actually increased enormously through sponsorship of major sporting events like the Benson and Hedges Cup in cricket and the Rothmans Tennis Tournament, events that have become synonymous with the sponsors' names. Newsagents can no longer display cigarette advertisements on their shop fronts for fear of enticing our children to become the smokers of tomorrow – or, more to the point, today. And yet, 64% of children in this country aged 9–15 see cigarette advertising on television while watching Grand Prix racing and the like. By using the cunning ploy of sponsoring sport on television, the tobacco industry has managed to sanitize its public image whilst, at the same time, widely publicizing its health-endangering products.

In 1990, in the USA, a move to break this artful mould was made by the Timberwolves, a Mid-West professional basketball team, when they made their arena a 'no smoking' zone in which all advertising and sale of tobacco products was prohibited. This was a brave step in a country in which professional sport is largely underpinned by funding from the tobacco industry. The Timberwolves' owners, who also run a health club at the ground, could no longer live with the contradiction inherent in the marriage of tobacco money with sport and health.

And yet, notwithstanding these trends towards a healthier, smoke-free world, smoking is still a most acceptable social habit. Princesses, politicians, doctors and film stars do it. Advertisements, where they are allowed, promote smoking as sexy and sophisticated. Young people, especially young women, are targeted and encouraged to start smoking by the tobacco industry's seductive message.

It was Christopher Columbus, his discoveries not limited to new continents, who first introduced tobacco to Europe in the fifteenth century. But the habit of smoking only took hold in the court of Elizabeth I a century later, having been initiated by Sir Francis Drake and Sir Walter Raleigh. Tobacco was considered to have miraculous healing powers; during the plague of London in 1665, Harrow schoolboys were compelled to smoke as a protective measure. Smoking cigarettes only became widespread when the technology was invented for their mass production at the turn of this century. At first it was for men only. But, after the First World War, women, having recently been given the vote and raised their hemlines, also started the smoking habit, no doubt as a further expression of their liberation.

Within twenty years, the link between cigarette smoking, heart disease and lung cancer had been established. Premature deaths were occurring in increasing numbers in smokers, initially in men and soon after in women as more of them took up the habit.

Today, 14 billion cigarettes are produced each day around the world. In the UK alone, tobacco produces an approximate income of

£15,500,000 per day. Although each packet of cigarettes carries a health warning and the government levies a 75% tax (estimated at £4 billion per year on cigarette sales), there are still 16 million smokers in this country. The tobacco industry makes £10 million each year from cigarettes sold illegally to children. There are 300 deaths each day from smoking; the tobacco industry needs to recruit 300 new smokers every day to replace them.

Smoking looks so harmless, so ordinary. It is a means of social bartering; it sets the scene. Offering someone a cigarette is perceived as a friendly gesture that can have any number of non-verbal connotations. To the suggestible youngsters of today, cigarette smoking is a life-style indicator along with Levi 501s and Carling Black Label.

The message that smoking is dangerous to our health has penetrated public conscious-ness to some extent; there are 11 million ex-smokers in the United Kingdom and 70% of those still smoking want to give it up. Many public places like tube trains, theatres and cinemas are no-smoking areas and attempts to catch the public's attention are made annually on No Smoking Day. Nevertheless, smoking continues to cause an epidemic of deaths many times worse than the most pessimistic projections of mortality due to AIDS in the twenty-first century.

A motorway pile-up or a train crash causing multiple fatalities hits the headlines and shocks and appals us – it could have been me, or you. The arbitrary nature of such deaths takes one's breath away. But 300 people dying of smoking-related diseases every day doesn't make the headlines.

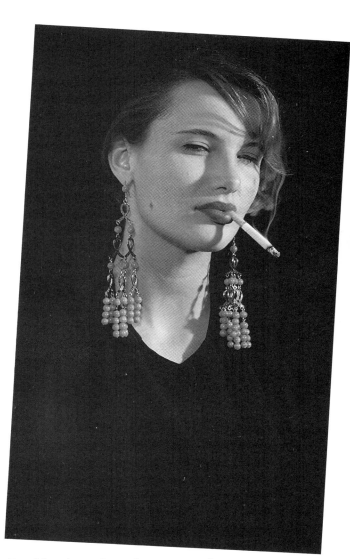

Smoking is portrayed as sexy and sophisticated by the tobacco industry

THE DEADLY FACTS ABOUT SMOKING:

* one person dies every thirteen seconds in the world from smoking

* one person dies every five minutes from smoking in the United Kingdom

* smoking kills 110,000 people in the United Kingdom each year

* a quarter of the people who smoke will die from smoking

* 40% of smokers die before reaching retirement age

* the average shortening of life is 10–15 years

* a cigarette smoker has nearly three times the risk of having a heart attack as a non-smoker

* 80% of heart attacks in men under forty-five are thought to be due to smoking cigarettes

* women smokers who take the pill run ten times the risk of having a heart attack or stroke than non-smoking non-pill takers

* smoking is responsible for at least 20% of deaths due to heart disease

* 90% of lung cancer and bronchitis deaths are due to smoking

* in EC countries, the commonest cancer in men is lung cancer; 95% of men with lung cancer are smokers

* smoking is the *largest single preventable cause of death*

Passive smoking

Passive smoking, in contradiction to its title, is something of a lively issue. Until fairly recently, non-smokers were very much the silent minority; even in a no-smoking railway carriage, they would hardly dare to challenge an oblivious smoker for fear of the miscreant's aggressive and humiliating rebuttal. Smokers definitely had the upper hand which they were not afraid of wielding, often tyrannically, over the muttering, grumbling, non-smokers. Lately though, the tables have turned somewhat since it has been confirmed that other people's smoke (sidestream smoke) with its lethal mixture of toxins and carcinogens can cause extreme physical harm. Armed with this ammunition, non-smokers of the world are uniting; they are finding their voice and standing up for their right to a healthy environment.

Many a row has been known to blow up in a family in which only one partner smokes, about who stays and who leaves the room during a favourite television programme. An hour spent in a poorly ventilated room, or worse still in a car, especially with a pipe- or cigar-smoker, can cause a non-smoker passively to inhale the equivalent amount of tobacco smoke inhaled from actively smoking one cigarette. Moreover, the concentration of harmful chemicals in sidestream smoke is higher than in the mainstream smoke inhaled through the cigarette by the smoker. Even so, smokers still tend to be treated like recalcitrant children who must be humoured to avoid a scene; I have known a whole party move outdoors and freeze so that the smoker amongst them should not feel an outcast. But the evidence is undeniable – passive smoking can kill!

Children as passive smokers

It would be horrifying to think of parents allowing a young child to smoke. And yet, parents who smoke expose their children to risks of contracting serious, often fatal, diseases. Children exposed to household cigarette smoke were found to be four times more likely to be admitted to hospital with serious infections such as meningitis, than children who had not been subjected to passive smoking. Another study found that cancer was more common by up to 30% in children whose parents smoked during pregnancy, even if the smoker was the father. One in every sixteen cases of all childhood cancers, in particular leukaemia, are linked with mothers smoking.

Recently, public consciousness has been raised concerning the dangers to health of nuclear radiation. The possible link between a

THE FACTS ABOUT PASSIVE SMOKING:

* Passive smoking causes lung cancer. In the United States, 3700 deaths a year are estimated to be due to lung cancer caused by passive smoking.

* Passive smoking is one of the major causes of heart disease.

* There is a 30% plus increased risk of death from heart disease in non-smoking spouses whose husbands or wives are smokers.

* The higher the cigarette consumption in the smoker, the higher the risk of heart disease in the non-smoking partner.

* In the United States, 53,000 deaths annually are attributed to passive smoking; 37,000 of these are from heart disease and 3700 from lung cancer.

* Non-smokers who have been exposed to other people's tobacco smoke throughout most of their life have a 10–30% higher risk of lung cancer than non-smokers who have not been so exposed.

father working at a nuclear plant like Sellafield and the existence of leukaemia years later in his offspring has raised the question of radiation causing a genetic defect in sperm cells. Rightly, this information has caused something of a furore. Less media attention has been paid to the specific association found between brain cancer in children and fathers smoking, which suggests that smoking can also cause a genetic defect in sperm cells.

The unborn babe as a passive smoker

Smoking is associated with about 9000 miscarriages a year and 450 perinatal baby deaths in Great Britain, some of which are due to low birth weight that reduces the baby's defence mechanisms and increases its vulnerability to infection, etc. Currently, only one in twelve women gives up smoking during pregnancy and two-thirds go back to cigarettes after the baby is born. If all pregnant women gave up cigarettes, the incidence of miscarriages could be halved and the rate of perinatal deaths cut by a quarter.

Why is tobacco smoke harmful?

Smoking and lung infection

Normal lungs have a very powerful and effective defence mechanism against the potentially damaging effects of bacteria and foreign material in the air to the delicate lining of the air-filled sacs. Tiny 'hairs', called cilia, exist on the surface of the lining cells that themselves produce mucus. The cilia and mucus together comprise a clearing mechanism, like a tide wafting any foreign substance or organism back up the air passages to the throat and, ultimately, the outside. In smokers, the mucus-clearing mechanism is slowed down causing damage to the lungs' defences so that bacteria can take hold and cause **chronic bronchitis** – the commonest cause of chronic illness, disability and absenteeism in this country.

Smoking and lung cancer

Tobacco smoke has nearly 4000 components which act as irritants to the lung tissue, causing damage to cells. **Cancer** is caused when certain of these irritant substances in the tar, which have carcinogenic properties, damage the genes (DNA) so that the wrong 'messages' get through and the cells behave in an abnormal, uncharacteristic fashion resulting in a malignant tumour.

The main tumour initiators in tobacco smoke are the N-nitrosamines. These compounds are also found in food and drink, but their intake is strictly controlled by government regulations. The upper limit allowed in food or drink is one part per billion. No such government regulations control the intake of these powerful cancer-causing agents in tobacco smoke, in which the concentration of N-nitrosamines ranges from 2000 to 9000 parts per billion.

Another of the cancer-producing substances is benzene. In 1990, the French mineral water company, Perrier, withdrew millions of bottles of their water from sale in response to public outcry when 4.7 microgrammes of benzene was found in some batches. Compare this with a single cigarette which contains up to 190 microgrammes of benzene.

WHY DON'T ALL SMOKERS GET CANCER?

For some cancers to develop there is thought to be a chain of causation consisting of the following three links:

1. A genetic predisposition to developing a specific cancer

2. A cancer-causing virus

3. A trigger – exposure to carcinogenic substances

If all three elements co-exist, whether in a smoker, or a non-smoker exposed to passive smoking, then the conditions are present for cancer to develop. This explains why some smokers may not get cancer, and non-smokers may do so.

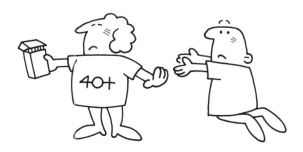

Smoking and heart disease

The substantially increased risk of heart disease in smokers is thought to be due to the fact that platelets in the blood become sticky and clump together at the sites of small 'wounds' in the arterial walls, causing the flow of blood to slow down which predisposes to the formation of blood clots. In the heart, these clots can cause coronary thrombosis, or **heart attacks**.

In the brain, they can cause **strokes**, and in the limbs, **gangrene**. It appears that the trigger is the nicotine in tobacco smoke which, as well as being a heart stimulant, releases the stress hormones, adrenalin and noradrenalin, causing vasoconstriction, or narrowing of the blood vessels.

The gases, carbon monoxide and nitrous oxide, found in cigarette smoke, can also lead to strokes, heart attacks and gangrene. In industry, government regulations forbid exposure to carbon monoxide levels over 50 parts per million. Tobacco smoke concentrations range from 1000 to 50,000 parts per million!

CIGAR AND PIPE SMOKING

It is a fallacy to imagine that, because pipe and cigar smoke are not inhaled, they carry no dangers to health. Although protected from the harmful effects of tobacco tar and gases, pipe- and cigar-smokers still take in a considerable amount of nicotine which, in cigar and pipe tobacco, is very soluble due to the way in which the tobacco is cured. The smoke only has to be held in the mouth (not inhaled into the lungs) for sufficient nicotine to be absorbed to have an effect. So, whilst pipe- and cigar-smokers are protected from the direct risks of lung cancer and chronic bronchitis, they are not immune to the effects of nicotine on the heart and circulatory systems – nor are their non-smoking friends and relations.

Smoking and duodenal ulcer

The incidence of duodenal ulcer is higher in smokers due to a decrease in secretions from the pancreas that normally buffer the acid from the stomach. As a result, the food being digested in the small intestine is more acid and can literally eat away at the duodenal wall, causing an ulcer.

Smoking and exercise

When oxygen and carbon monoxide are both present in inhaled air, carbon monoxide has a more than 100 times better chance of bonding with the oxygen-carrying haemoglobin in the blood than oxygen. In average individuals, this oxygen lack is pretty immaterial; but in endurance athletes it is very serious as the amount of oxygen reaching the working muscles, including the heart, may be inadequate. A smoker engaging in vigorous endurance exercise should not smoke for at least four hours beforehand as this is the time taken for carbon monoxide reasonably to clear from the blood. Furthermore, anyone taking part in strenuous exercise should avoid both smoking and alcohol for at least half an hour after stopping, because the heart muscle is particularly sensitive to fibrillation during that

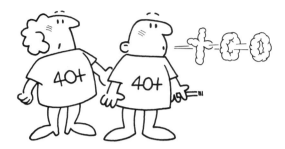

period. There is a message here for the lunch-time squash player who, after a game, just has time for a beer and a cigarette before rushing back to his or her next meeting.

Smoking and addiction

Nicotine is a highly addictive drug that creates physical and psychological dependence. Smokers who try to stop often experience withdrawal symptoms, including craving, irritability, anxiety, reduced concentration, restlessness, headache and gastro-intestinal disturbances. If you are a hardened smoker, you will know how important is the first cigarette of the morning. If you do not get your fix, you start to feel all those withdrawal symptoms mentioned above. Within seven seconds of inhaling that first drag, nicotine is detectable in the brain cells. The effect is felt all over the body within nineteen seconds, almost as fast as if the drug had been injected intravenously. You continue to smoke during the day to stop any further withdrawal symptoms which you would otherwise feel.

Smokers think cigarettes make them feel good but, in fact, they are simply preventing them from feeling bad. The addiction is to the nicotine, but it is, for the most part, the carbon monoxide and tar that do the mortal damage.

First steps in kicking the habit

Smoking is a complex habit and behaviour
pattern. People smoke for a variety of effects.
Which category do you fall into? Do you:

* smoke after meals to relax?

* need something to do with your hands?

* smoke to improve concentration when
  working?

* light up out of habit, automatically?

* smoke to alleviate stress in stressful situations?

* smoke because everyone else does?

The first thing to discover is how much you
really want to stop smoking. If you are not
truly committed to stopping you may simply
reinforce your belief that you cannot stop. It is
helpful in the first instance to discover why
you smoke. Do you smoke in social situations
where you feel relaxed? Or are you more likely
to smoke when you feel angry, miserable or
stressed? Some people use cigarettes to relieve
unpleasant feelings, while others smoke to
enhance their enjoyment. In all smokers,
stress-management techniques, like simple
relaxation, would be a helpful strategy for
coping with stressful situations when the
compulsion to smoke is greatest.

Although 90% of the 11 million ex-smokers
in Great Britain stopped smoking without any
special support, you may be one of the many
smokers for whom stopping smoking has not
become a reality. Although you have accepted
the health education messages that smoking is
harmful, you are unable to take the next decis-
ive step towards giving up. It is now recog-
nized that stopping smoking is not one single
simple event. It is a process that requires
many changes in both attitude and behaviour.

It begins when the smoker first feels some
doubts about the habit and recognizes that it is
an addiction. The intention to stop smoking
follows on from this realization, as a result of
which smokers may no longer be happy about

continuing with their habit. Nevertheless, many do not yet feel ready or able to stop. It is at this point that help and support may well be needed. Many GPs are now holding clinics to help people stop smoking. Also, a number of other private organizations run workshops to help smokers kick the habit. These workshops encourage people to succeed by helping them to develop these three attitudes:

* *confidence* in your ability to give up smoking

* *determination* to deal with withdrawal symptoms of nicotine

* *motivation* to stop smoking by focusing on the reasons and advantages like health, cost, responsibility to one's children, concern for others and the environment

As with any habit-forming drug, the first two weeks of withdrawal of nicotine are usually the worst. At this point, it is useful to keep two messages in mind.

* *smoking is a killer*

* *stopping smoking does you good!*

Many people believe that, having smoked for many years, there is little point in giving up smoking, because they are already at risk of developing one or other of the serious and often fatal diseases that their habit causes. Others believe that since they are not suffering from any of these diseases at the present moment, they are in some way or other immune. Here are the facts:

* The more years you smoke and the greater the number of cigarettes smoked daily, the greater the risk to your health; the onset of disease can start at any time.

* The good news is that ten years after stopping smoking, your risk of heart attack and lung cancer is reduced to that of a life-long non-smoker. The benefits from not smoking start to accrue the *moment that you stop*.

How can you stop smoking?

In 1988 the World Health Organisation, in collaboration with the International Union against Cancer, issued guidelines relating to the four stages of stopping smoking: thinking about stopping, preparing to stop, stopping and staying 'stopped'.

A strategy is needed:

1. Decide on a stopping date. Write it down, enter it in your diary.

2. Write down all your reasons for stopping and have these near at hand as a reminder when the going gets tough.

3. Go public – tell your family, friends, colleagues and enlist their support.

4. Pair up with a friend prepared to stop smoking on the same day and keep in touch with each other's progress.

5. Practise saying, 'I don't smoke,' when offered cigarettes.

6. Distract yourself – fiddle with worry beads or chew gum.

7. Remove all cigarettes from your home, car and place of work.

8. If weight gain is your fear – read the chapters on nutrition and diet, weight-control and exercise. Armed with this information, engage in a programme of exercise and sensible eating to avoid weight gain.

9. If you fail and start smoking again, consider the reasons why, what the pressures were and how to cope with these in the future. Then set another stopping date and try again.

HELP WITH BREAKING THE HABIT

Nicotine gum is a good substitute if your craving for nicotine is unbearable. Take a piece of gum when you feel the urge to smoke a cigarette and keep it in the mouth for 20–30 minutes, chewing it every minute or so to get the effect of absorbed nicotine. After three months without smoking your use of the gum should be gradually reduced.

Nicotine nasal spray may also be a successful way to wean yourself off smoking, but it may also be highly addictive. Nicotine skin patches are also being tested.

Herbal cigarettes are thought to be a good alternative for smokers wishing to break the nicotine habit, but herbal cigarettes are, themselves, dangerous to health, because they too contain tar and produce carbon monoxide gas.

Hypnosis and acupuncture have been shown to be useful in helping some smokers to quit.

A FINAL WORD

If warnings about the risks of cancer, heart disease and early death are not effective in persuading you to give up smoking perhaps vanity might be.

Smoking causes wrinkles! Smoking may help you to keep your weight down, but the price you pay may be premature ageing. Smokers are nearly five times more likely to be heavily wrinkled than non-smokers.

Smokers lose their teeth! Smoking can cause loss of bone around the teeth, so that they are likely to fall out.

Not a pretty sight!

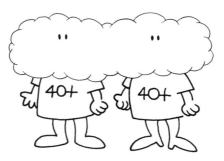

FIVE

Food Glorious Food

The human body is a bit like the *Queen Elizabeth II* – not HM, but SS – a powerhouse, a city complete in itself, with everything aboard for the survival and comfort of its passengers and crew as it cruises the high seas from one port to the next, its engines silently and ceaselessly throbbing. Even when in dock (sleeping?), the work carries on as it is repaired, renewed and refitted ready to sail full-steam ahead on its next voyage.

There are two kinds of things that are needed in order for the vessel to remain in tip-top condition and to maintain its reputation as the greatest cruise ship ever to put to sea. First, materials and supplies; materials to refit and replace where wear-and-tear has taken its toll, and supplies to fulfil every need of the passengers and crew. Second, it needs fuel to get it from continent to continent, plus another kind of energy, manpower, to ensure its smooth and efficient running.

The human body needs building materials and energy to grow, develop and maintain itself, for organs to function effectively, for tissue growth, renewal, repair and regeneration, for the millions of chemical reactions to take place both inside and outside the cells, for the action of the muscles in physical activity, and to maintain body temperature. The food we eat supplies both the building materials and the energy so that the body can sustain this process of life.

Food glorious food – there's nothing quite like it. Not only is food essential for life, it is also one of life's greatest pleasures, titillating the senses with its taste, colour, smell and texture. By its appearance and presentation, food stimulates our brain and nervous system; the appetite is whetted and the gastric juices flow. Like sex, food satisfies a basic human need while providing comfort and gratification.

But, although your brain tells you what you like to eat and drink, its selection may not always be in your body's best interests. Habit and cultural mores may play a significant part – for instance, fish on Fridays and Christmas pudding at Christmas. Also, past associations from childhood, like being comforted with sweets and chocolate when injured or upset, can establish a life-long pattern of turning to sugary foods when miserable or sad.

Once inside the body, the role food plays changes to one of providing nourishment. The value of the food we eat can be assessed

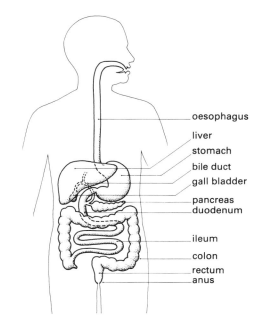

Figure 4   The digestive system

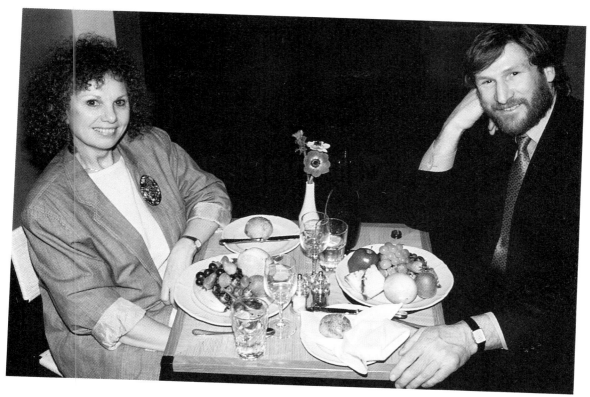

Liz and Andy with a healthy snack!

by breaking it down into its components, called *nutrients*, as happens in the digestive system. In order to remain healthy, the body needs nearly fifty essential nutrients which can *only* be obtained from the food we eat. These nutrients include carbohydrates, fats, proteins, dietary fibre, vitamins, minerals, trace elements and water. By varying the amount and type of food you eat, you can adjust the relative proportions of the various nutrients in your diet – you can have a high-protein diet, a low-fat diet, a low-salt diet, a high-carbohydrate/low-fat diet, a high-fibre diet and so on.

Nutrients also supply the energy or fuel needed for all the body's processes, chemical reactions and physical activity. After food is digested the component nutrients are absorbed into the blood in a useable form and carried around the body to organs and tissues where they are utilized. If the energy available from the food is more than is being used up by the body, the excess is stored as fat – like in a larder.

What is a healthy diet?

This is not an easy question to answer. Before even attempting it, we need to clarify some of the confusing gobbledegook that has accumulated around words like 'diet'. Each week, four or five books about weight-loss appear in the bestseller list, all of them having the word 'diet' in their titles. Consequently, the word 'diet' has become synonymous with eating plans, the aim of which is to lose weight. In fact, your diet is your everyday pattern of food intake.

There are good diets and poor diets. At one end of the spectrum, there are the well-composed, balanced diets that provide adequate essential nutrients and energy for the nutrition process to do its job properly, resulting in good health. At the other end, there are the appallingly deficient starvation diets that 27 million Ethiopians and Sudanese are currently enduring. Somewhere in the middle, in nutritional terms, are the faddy, fanciful diets in which we in the West are prone to indulge, diets associated with promises of weight-loss – the egg and grapefruit diet . . . the pineapple and pomegranate diet . . . the drinking man's diet . . . the yoghurt and banana diet – that are deficient in energy and also some essential nutrients.

During the post-war rationing period the diet in the UK, devoid of treats and trimmings, was actually healthier than the high-fat/high-sugar diet typical of the more prosperous years that followed.

Regional diets typical of people living in a certain country have evolved largely as a result of the local availability of plants, vegetables and animals. The nature of these food sources is itself largely dependent on the geographical location, climate, soil and water supply. Beans are a staple food in the Mexican diet because more than fifty varieties are grown there. The Eskimo diet consists mainly of fish, seal and whale meat which are readily available to the Inuit (to the exclusion of much else), whilst the principal constituent of the diet in the Indian sub-continent is rice.

Dietary patterns have emerged regionally from food sources which are easily grown, sown and produced, but with little knowledge

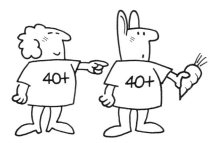

of food composition, although the medicinal, therapeutic and curative properties of particular plants like herbs have been known since the first civilizations. There is a huge variety of different diets eaten by people throughout the world and with the different diets come a host of different disease patterns. It would be impossible to point a finger at a particular population living in some isolated corner of the globe and say they had the perfect, healthy diet. But knowledge gained in two fields of scientific research has given us clues as to the possible nature of healthy eating; they are studies of

1. Nutrition

2. Diet and associated disease

Nutrition – what is it?

Nutrition refers to the processes in the body that utilize the food eaten to provide the essential nutrients and energy we need to survive. The study of nutrition is the science of food – it tells us what is in food and what happens to it in the body.

Table 3
Examples of foods rich in dietary fibre

The figures show how many grams of fibre each item contains, and apply to one average-sized portion (unless otherwise stated).

All-Bran	8.5	peanuts (unsalted, 30 g)	2
apple, small	2	pear	4
large	4	peas	7
apricots, 3 medium	1.4	plantain	5
2 dried	7	porridge	3
banana	3	potatoes, baked in jacket	3
barley (cooked)	3	boiled with skin	3
baked beans	6	boiled without skin	1
blackberries (100 g)	3.3	prunes, 3 dried	4.7
bread (per slice), brown	1.5	Puffed Wheat	4
chapati	0.75	raisins (30 g)	2
white	0.75	rice, brown	3
wholemeal	2.75	white	2
broccoli (cooked)	2.8	Shredded Wheat (2)	5
carrots (cooked)	3.2	spaghetti, ordinary	2
cornflakes	3	wholemeal	6
dahl	3	spinach	5
figs, 3 dried	7.2	sprouts	2
kidney beans (red, cooked)	9.3	swede	2
leeks	3	sweetcorn	5
lentils	4	strawberries (200 g)	2.8
muesli (unsugared)	4	Weetabix (2)	5
oat bran	5.5	yam	3
peach	1.3		

THE BUILDING BLOCKS

Carbohydrates are the main source of energy in most diets.

Simple carbohydrates, or sugars, are found in fruit, milk and cane sugar, maple syrup, etc. Refined sugar occurs in large quantities in highly processed sweet foods like sweets, confectionery, jams and soft drinks.

Sugar is rapidly absorbed and requires little digestion, so it is a source of instant energy, but it contains *nothing* of nutritious value in the way of vitamins, minerals, trace elements and fibre. Sugary foods are a cause of dental decay. In addition, sugar is often combined with a lot of fat in foods like pies, cakes, biscuits and puddings to provide a great many calories but little else, contributing to overweight and a diet deficient in vitamins and minerals.

Complex carbohydrates – starchy foods – are the most widespread form of carbohydrate in the plant world and are found in seeds, grains and cereals (from which bread and pasta are made), rice, peas, beans, potatoes, nuts and vegetables. They are best eaten in their natural, unrefined state in which, in addition to their high energy content, they supply essential vitamins and minerals, together with dietary fibre.

Starches and sugars are broken down in the gut to glucose and absorbed into the blood stream as blood glucose which is then readily available to meet the body's high demand for energy, particularly in the brain where it is the *only* source of energy that can be used and is essential for normal brain function. Excess carbohydrates can be stored for future use, either as glycogen in the liver and muscle or as fat in fat deposits. Carbohydrates provide 4 Kcal energy per gram.

Dietary fibre is the indigestible cellulose portion of grains, cereals, vegetables and fruit. During the past century, our diet has contained diminishing amounts of fibre – a decrease that is associated with an increase in a number of chronic medical conditions, including cancer of the colon, high blood cholesterol, diabetes and coronary heart disease. A healthy diet should be high in fibre, with a daily intake of 25–35g (see Table 3).

Fats can be found in both plant and animal food sources. They can be classified as 'visible' fats (butter, lard, cooking oil, etc.) which contribute 30% or more to the normal daily fat intake, or 'invisible' as in meat, eggs, cheese, milk, nuts, vegetables and cereals, which account for the remaining 70%.

Fat in animal food sources (meat, cheese, milk, eggs) is **saturated** (a reference to its chemical structure), whilst that in plants is **unsaturated**. In the West, animal fats make up about two-thirds of our fat intake, and fat from vegetables (oils such as sunflower-seed oil, peanut oil, etc.) the other third. Whilst fat in the diet is essential in order to remain healthy, health agencies (e.g. World Health Organisation) currently recommend a significant reduction in total fat intake to 30% or less of total calories with animal fat making up only 10% of total calories. These recommendations are made in order to reduce the incidence of heart disease, certain cancers, hypertension, obesity and gall stones.

Fats provide the largest store of energy in the body, protect vital organs and insulate

Table 4
The fat content of some common foods

The figures show how many grams of fat each item contains, and apply to one average-sized portion (unless otherwise stated).

bacon, streaky (60g) fried	25	fish fingers (3), fried	11
grilled	20	grilled	6
burger ¼lb	20	ghee (10g)	10
butter or margarine (10g)	8	halva	11
low-fat spread	4	liver (60g) fried	8
chapati (made with fat)	10	stewed	6
Cheddar cheese (60g)	19	mince (85g)	14
low fat	9	with fat poured off	6
chicken (85g) roast with skin	12	paratha	22
roast without skin	4	peanuts (small bag)	12
Chinese pastry with bean filling	6	pork chop (85g)	
chips, thin cut	17	fried with fat on	25
thick cut	8	grilled with fat on	20
oven	7	grilled with fat removed	8
chocolate, small bar	15	pork pie	30
cod (85g), fried in batter	9	potatoes, baked/boiled	0.1
steamed	1	roast	8
cottage cheese (60g)	2	samosa (1)	26
cream/yoghurt (30g), double	13	sausages (2 large)	21
single	6	low fat	11
low-fat yoghurt	0.3	steak (85g)	
crisps (small bag)	9	grilled, lean and fat	20
low fat	7	grilled, lean only	8
digestive biscuits (2)	6	steak and kidney pie	24
Edam cheese (60g)	13		

from the cold. They also act as carriers of the fat-soluble vitamins – A, D, E and K. During light to moderate exercise, fat provides about half the energy required. In heavy, prolonged work, more than 80% of the energy needs come from fat stores. Fat provides 9 Kcal of energy per gram.

Cholesterol is present in all cells of the body and is either eaten in certain foods – egg yolks, red organ meat and shellfish – or made within the cells. It is essential for a number of chemical processes including the secretion of sex hormones and the formation of bile in the liver.

Protein is found in all food as it exists in the cells of all animals and plants. Protein is made up of amino acids – the body needs twenty of these to be healthy, nine of which (called essential amino acids) cannot be made in the body and must be supplied in the diet.

Animal proteins found in meat, cheese, fish, poultry, milk and eggs contain all nine essential amino acids in the correct ratio and are called high quality complete proteins because they can be used as the building materials for tissue growth and repair. Vegetable protein in beans, lentils, peas, nuts, seeds and cereals is incomplete because it lacks one or more of the essential amino acids. However, a vegetarian can have a complete protein diet by eating a *variety* of vegetable foods (including all the above plus wholegrains, brown rice and soya) which, together, provide all the essential amino acids. Two-thirds of the world's population are adequately nourished on a varied vegetarian diet with only a small amount of protein. Protein provides 4 Kcal of energy per gram, although it is not primarily an *energy* source.

OUR NUTRITIONAL NEEDS

Each food has a nutrient content and an energy value. For example, the nutrient content of 100g of Cheddar cheese is 26g protein, 35g fat (of which 22g is saturated fat), and its energy value is 410 Kcal.

Individuals vary in their requirements for various nutrients according to their state of health and physical activity. For a diet to be healthy, it needs to be composed of correct proportions of nutrients for a particular individual.

For example

* A woman endurance athlete needs a higher calorie intake (say 3000 Kcal per day if she trains for fifty miles per week) than her less active sister who needs about 2000 Kcal per day. The athlete may also need food rich in iron and calcium as these can become depleted with stamina training.

* Women taking an oral contraceptive may need extra vitamins B1, B2, B6 and C and folic acid as these tend to be depleted in women taking the pill.

* Smoking reduces the body's vitamin C so smokers need to take in extra to make up for this.

* Excess alcohol intake may impair absorption of vitamin B1, folic acid, B12 and C, so food particularly rich in these vitamins is needed.

*   Children and women (particularly during pregnancy, lactation and when post-meno-pausal) need extra calcium; in children and pregnant or lactating women to help build strong bones, and in post-menopausal women, to limit the loss of bone that occurs when oestrogen levels drop and which predisposes to osteoporosis and bone fractures.

People with specific medical conditions need special diets. For instance, a person with kidney disease requires a diet much lower in protein than is normal, because his or her kidneys are unable to deal with the nitrogen-based waste products of protein. These toxic waste products are life endangering to the kidney-disease sufferer – a true case of one man's meat poisoning another. But this diet would contain an inadequate and unhealthy proportion of protein for a healthy individual. Individuals involved in specific activities have particular dietary needs: a marathon runner may eat a diet high in complex carbohydrate – pasta, rice, etc. – for two or three days before the race (a procedure called carbohydrate-loading) to create high reserves of glycogen in the muscles.

Paradoxically, it is possible to be overfed and yet poorly nourished, a condition not uncommonly found in the West, where large amounts of heavily refined, fast or junk food have replaced the unprocessed, whole, nutrient-rich food typical of more underdeveloped regions of the world. The result is a diet deficient in essential nutrients.

Table 5 Calcium content of some common foods

	mg calcium/ 100mg food	Kcal
almonds	250	565
apple	4	40
bread, brown and white	100	223
Brussel sprouts	25	18
Cheddar cheese	810	391
double cream	50	447
egg, whole	56	160
fig, dried	280	213
haddock	55	98
milk, skimmed	120	35
milk, whole	120	66
Parmesan cheese	1290	379
parsley	330	21
potatoes, baked in skins	9	85
potatoes, boiled	4	80
rhubarb	100	6
single cream	80	212
spinach	600	30
spring greens	86	10
tomatoes	11	14
walnuts	61	525
watercress	220	14
whitebait, fried	860	525
yoghurt, low fat	143	39

Recommended dietary allowance of calcium (daily amounts in mg)

Children		500–1000
Women:		500–1000
	pregnant	1000–2000
	breast feeding	1000–2000
Men		500– 800

Diet and associated disease

HIGH-FAT DIET

The typical Western diet of today is high fat (especially animal fats), high sugar (refined in sweets, cakes, confectionery, etc.) and low fibre – a diet which promotes the chronic diseases associated with the adult populations in Western developed countries:

* heart disease

* high blood pressure

* obesity

* diabetes

* various cancers (breast, uterus, prostate)

* gall bladder disease

It was not always this way.

While technology has definitely led to progress, it has also brought us food refining and processing that have resulted in food in which essential minerals, vitamins and fibre have been lost, e.g. polished rice is minus the valuable husk on the outer surface; this lack in populations whose diets are largely dependent on rice, can cause beriberi, a deficiency disease due to lack of vitamin B1. More recently, the common practice of adding artificial colouring, flavouring and preservatives to food has been associated with allergic conditions. During the past two decades, the in-

vasive spread of fast-food and junk-food outlets all over the world has been phenomenally fast. A 1000-calorie fast-food meal consisting of a hamburger, french fries and a milk shake epitomizes the high-fat/high-sugar diet common today in the Western world; not only does it provide an excess of calories but more than 60% of those calories are from animal fat which raises the blood cholesterol level.

High blood cholesterol seriously increases the risk of coronary heart disease, particularly if combined with other risk factors like cigarette-smoking, obesity and hypertension; the risk is greater in men than in pre-menopausal women whose oestrogen levels give them protection. A change of diet is the first line of treatment in a person with high blood cholesterol, not only to reduce the levels of fat in the blood, but also to produce a desirable weight-loss.

The recommended dietary changes to reduce cholesterol levels are:

1. Total fat intake reduced to 30% or less of total dietary calorie intake.

2. Saturated fats (animal fat, hydrogenated vegetable oils) reduced to 10% of total and partially replaced with mono-unsaturated (e.g. olive oil) and polyunsaturated fatty acids (vegetable oils such as sunflower-seed, corn and nut oils).

3. Cholesterol intake reduced to less than 300 milligrams per day (by limiting animal fat). See Table 6, page 54.

4. More complex carbohydrates to replace the

A healthy diet is one that meets the nutritional needs of a particular individual according to his or her state of health and physical activity.

calories lost from eating less fat (fruits, vegetables and cereal fibre plus pulses and legumes).

5. Alcohol intake reduced to moderate only, i.e., recommended levels: up to 21 units per week for men and 14 units per week for women (see page 63).

6. Sugar intake reduced to less than 10% of total dietary calories.

7. Fish, especially salmon, tuna, sardines and halibut, as often as you like but at least 2–3 times a week.

Despite its bad reputation, cholesterol does have a number of important functions to perform in the body, including manufacturing sex hormones and bile salts. It is only when the levels of cholesterol in the blood are high that its bad reputation is deserved, because then it tends to accumulate in the walls of arteries causing, in the course of time, narrowing of these vessels and atherosclerosis. It is the narrowing of the *coronary* arteries supplying the heart muscle that can eventually lead to a total blockage of these vessels and possibly a fatal heart attack. Reducing cholesterol levels in the blood is a necessary first step in avoiding heart disease; the most effective approach, however, is through a combination of diet and exercise.

A programme of aerobic exercise, i.e., exercise sufficient to raise the heart rate and make you a little breathless, is strongly recommended both to reduce the total blood cholesterol levels and to help weight-loss. In addition, regular physical exercise produces a shift in the ratio of the two sorts of cholesterol with the so-called 'bad' low-density lipoprotein portion (LDL) levels decreasing and the 'good' high-density lipoprotein portion (HDL) increasing.

Breast cancer has been linked with a high-fat diet which, in turn, is associated with high oestrogen levels. Women who reduce their fat intake to 20% of total calories in the diet produce a significant lowering of hormone levels accompanied by a drop in blood cholesterol and loss of weight.

Blood cholesterol is raised considerably by drinking coffee made by mixing coffee grounds with boiling water, whereas filtered

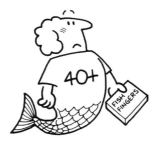

Table 6
Amount of dietary cholesterol in some sample foods

Food	mg of cholesterol per oz (unless otherwise stated)
egg yolk	250 per yolk
herring roe, soft, fried	200
lamb's kidney, fried	170
paste, chicken liver	120
sweetbreads	110
beef liver, fried	95
shrimp/prawn	25
mussels	20

coffee (in which the water is poured on to grounds in a paper filter through which the coffee drips into a jug) produces only a negligible rise. Anyone wishing to lower their blood cholesterol should avoid drinking boiled coffee.

Garlic is being promoted by scientists as having an important role to play in heart disease as a cholesterol-lowering agent, as well as in the prevention of cancer due to its anti-bacterial and anti-fungal activity.

Dietary cholesterol is high in foods that include eggs, offal and shellfish.

HIGH SUGAR INTAKE

Sugar in its refined form – like the sugar you put in your tea – contains nothing of use to your body except calories. British people have the sweetest tooth in Europe, consuming an average of 80 lbs of sugar per person each year, two-thirds of which comes in processed foods like biscuits, cakes, sweets, soft drinks and jam. Sugar in these foods is harmful to health because it promotes

* *tooth decay* by encouraging the bacteria on teeth to produce acid that eats away at the tooth enamel.

* *obesity*. It is easy to eat too many calories as sugar, because (i) sweet foods are low in fibre and fail to create a satisfied full feeling and (ii) sweet foods paradoxically create a desire to eat more. Initially, digested sugar quickly results in a high level of blood glucose. But the body's response is a surge of insulin that causes the blood sugar to take a dive. The result is hypoglycaemia (low blood-sugar level) with weakness, light-headedness and fatigue, and a desire to compensate with more sweet food.

Contrary to the popular belief in 'instant energy', sugar, sweets or glucose should not be eaten just before exercising because of this rebound insulin effect. *During* exercise, it is a different story. Exercise inhibits the release of insulin and taking in glucose in the form of a glucose drink *during* exercise is to be encouraged.

Craving for sweets is not uncommon; the symptoms of premenstrual tension are made worse in women who experience this kind of craving and succumb by bingeing on simple carbohydrates.

Sugar comes in a number of forms – sucrose, dextrose, fructose and maltose – and is also found in savoury foods like baked beans and soup. As well as seeing these forms of sugar listed on packaged food labels you may also find honey, syrup, raw sugar, brown sugar and muscovado which, while sounding healthy, are simply sugar in disguise.

Breakfast cereals, cereal bars and muesli may be hiding large amounts of sugar under their healthy food image; oats are almost unpalatable without some sugar and fat (unless you are a hardy Scot brought up on plain porridge); carrot cake, one imagines, must be healthy, otherwise surely no one would ever have thought of putting carrots in a cake when there are yummy things like cream, chocolate and strawberries to choose from. But its high sugar and oil content is lethal to anyone monitoring their health and waistline. Reading food labels is time well spent if a healthy diet is your goal.

Fruit is almost completely sugar (fructose) but, unlike refined sugar, it comes in combination with health-giving vitamins, minerals, trace elements and fibre. Whole fruit is preferable to fruit juice because the pectin in the whole fruit slows down the release of fruit sugar into the blood.

SALT IN THE DIET

On average we eat the equivalent of two whole teaspoonsful of salt daily, more than half of which is in processed food. Salt is naturally present in food and most people do not need more than a fifth of a teaspoon, which is the merest pinch, per day.

In people with hypertension, reducing dietary salt intake lowers blood pressure. If the salt added by food manufacturers to processed foods were reduced, it is estimated that deaths from strokes and coronary heart disease would be reduced by up to 40%, due to a significant reduction in blood pressure in the population as a whole. This is equivalent to preventing 65,000 deaths a year in Britain.

THE ESKIMO DIET – VERY FISHY!

Eskimos living in North-west Greenland eat a traditional diet of fish, seal and caribou; they also have a very low incidence of atherosclerosis (hardening of the arteries). Their brother and sister Eskimos who have migrated to Denmark, however, and eat a standard Western diet, suffer from coronary heart disease to the same extent as native Danes. In Japan, it was found that the cause of death in fish-eating fishermen was rarely due to heart disease whereas Japanese farmers who eat more animal fat commonly died of this condition. From these studies, the idea emerged that a high-fish diet may be the explanation for the apparent immunity of fish-eaters to fatal heart disease. Research has subsequently revealed that it is the *particular polyunsaturated fatty acids* (eicosapentaenoic acid – EPA, and docosahexanoic acid – DHA) that help prevent heart disease by

* lowering the levels of total cholesterol

* lowering the levels of LDL cholesterol

* raising the levels of HDL cholesterol

* helping prevent the formation of thrombosis and clots in the blood vessels

* reducing blood viscosity so it flows more easily

* having an anti-inflammatory effect

All of these effects inhibit the processes that lead to atherosclerosis and protect against arterial narrowing and coronary heart disease.

Due to the anti-inflammatory effect of EPA, fish oil has proved beneficial in the treatment of rheumatoid arthritis, asthma and psoriasis. High levels of EPA also exist, more exotically, in snake oil, capsules of which have been prescribed in this country as an arthritis cure.

HIGH-FIBRE DIET

In the past the wholefood, healthfood lobby which zealously promoted the benefits of eating high-fibre foods, had many detractors among the orthodox. Their claims were pooh-poohed as the quasi-religious ravings of sockless, sandal-wearing cranks. Recently, however, the arbiters of medical opinion have had to eat their hats (as well as their fibre). It is now known that low-fibre diets are associated with the development of a number of medical conditions, especially coronary heart disease, some cancers, e.g. colon and rectum, diabetes, diverticulosis and gall stones. High levels of dietary fibre, on the other hand, have therapeutic and protective effects in these medical conditions.

Fibre is the indigestible fraction of plant and vegetable foods. There are two types of fibre:

1. Bulking agents which are water insoluble and act by decreasing the time that food spends in the gut. The result of this hastened journey is that carcinogens in the biproducts of digested food in the gut, such as the nitrosamines, traces of which can be found in red meat and smoked, pickled and salt-cured food, spend less time in contact with the lining of the intestine and have less chance of detrimentally affecting the cells lining the walls.

   Good food sources of these bulking-type fibres include root and leafy vegetables, wholegrains (such as wheat, barley, rice and oats), legumes, unpeeled apples and pears, and strawberries.

2. Water-soluble fibre that has the ability to lower cholesterol levels by binding with the cholesterol in bile in the gut and preventing it from being recycled back into the body's pool. It is also effective in slowing down and reducing the blood-sugar rise that normally occurs after a sugar-rich meal and which can cause an insulin kick-back followed by rebound low blood-sugar known as hypoglycaemia.

   Good food sources of water-soluble fibre include barley, rice, corn, oats, legumes, apples and pears (the fleshy bits), citrus fruits, bananas, carrots, prunes, cranberries and seeds. Oat bran is particularly effective whereas wheat bran is not.

The average Western diet contains inadequate fibre – only about ten grams per day. Ideally, the fibre content should be two or three times this amount. Dietary fibre can be increased by eating a higher proportion of un-refined starchy foods and fruit and veget-ables. These foods are also low in fat and have a high level of many vitamins and minerals, factors that are known to offer protection against many chronic diseases. High-fibre foods have an important place in the WHO 1990s recommended eating plan (see page 60).

But, resist the temptation to *supplement* your diet with *refined* fibre as your absorption of essential minerals, such as calcium, iron, zinc and others, may be seriously diminished as a result. Obtaining fibre only from food in the diet makes it difficult to consume too much.

VITAMINS IN THE DIET

While fruit and vegetables, along with the starchy, wholefood carbohydrates, contribute greatly to the intake of dietary fibre, they also have other qualities that add considerably to their health value. They contain an abundance of antioxidants – vitamins A, C, E and beta-carotene – that mop up harmful free radicals in the cells before they have the chance to do any damage; DNA remains intact and unharmed, and tumours may be prevented from develop-ing. (See pages 25-27.)

It appears that vitamins increase the im-munological response in the body to tackle abnormal cell production. Studies on people with high levels of beta-carotene and vitamin A show that they have half the risk of dev-eloping cancer of the oesophagus compared to the general population.

Vitamin C may protect against stomach and gastrointestinal cancers. Applied to the skin, it gives protection against UV radiation damage that can cause skin cancer.

Vitamin E is considered to be a protective agent in heart disease, especially when com-bined with vitamin C. People with low levels of vitamin E and C have three times the in-cidence of angina, even excluding smokers who have low vitamin C due to smoking. How do E and C act as protectors?

High blood cholesterol, which is associated with narrowing of the coronary arteries and, in turn, with angina, has to be in an oxidized form to accumulate in the coronary arterial walls. Adequate supplies of antioxidant vitamins E and C will prevent cholesterol being oxidized. But lack of these antioxidants will result in oxidized cholesterol accumulat-ing and causing angina.

To reduce the risks of coronary heart disease and cancer the daily diet should con-tain an abundance of

* *vitamin E foods*

   cereals

   legumes

   vegetable oils; corn, sunflower, etc

* *vitamin C and vitamin A foods*

   dark green, leafy vegetables – broccoli, cabbage, kohlrabi

   yellow fruit and vegetables – mangos, apri-cots, carrots, swedes

   potatoes, apples, pears, berries

Table 7 Vitamins and minerals

Vitamins	Recommended Daily Intake (mg)	Best Dietary Sources	Effects of Deficiency	Effects of Excess
Water-soluble				
Vitamin B-1 (Thiamine)	1.5	dried brewer's yeast, pork, liver, wholegrains, brown rice, legumes, nuts, wheatgerm, soya flour, oatflakes	fatigue, muscle weakness, loss of appetite, nausea, digestive upsets, beriberi if deficiency excessive (rare in Europe)	none reported
Vitamin B-2 (Riboflavin)	1.8	widely distributed in foods – liver, wheatgerm, dairy products	inflamed tongue and lips, cracks at corner of mouth, lesions of eye	none reported
Niacin	20	liver, lean meats, grains, legumes, yeast extract, dried brewer's yeast, wheatbran, nuts, soya flour	pellagra – dermatitis, diarrhoea and dementia	flushing, burning and tingling around neck, face and hands, dry skin
Vitamin B-6 (Pyridoxine)	2	meats, vegetables, wholegrain cereals, bananas, nuts	irritability, depression, breast discomfort, skin complaints, kidney stones	neurological symptoms reported occasionally only if more than 200mg taken per day for a year or more
Pantothenic Acid	5-10	widely distributed in foods – liver, kidney, nuts, soya flour, wheatbran, wholegrains	fatigue, sleep disturbances, depression, headaches, aching, throbbing feet, loss of appetite, indigestion	none reported
Folacin (Folic Acid)	0.4	soya flour, wheatgerm, legumes, green vegetables, wholegrains, nuts	anaemia, weakness, fatigue, irritability, insomnia, confusion	only reported if more than 15mg daily taken: nausea, loss of appetite, gastrointestinal disturbances
Vitamin B-12	0.003	muscle and organ meats, fish, eggs, dairy products (not present in plant foods)	pernicious anaemia, smooth, sore tongue, neurological disorders, weakness, fatigue	none reported
Biotin	Not estab-lished.*	legumes, vegetables, meats	fatigue, depression, nausea, dermatitis, muscle pains	none reported
Choline	Not estab-lished.**	egg yolk, liver, lecithin, grains, legumes (all foods containing phospholipids)	none reported	none reported
Vitamin C (Ascorbic Acid)	45-60	citrus fruits, rosehip syrup, tomatoes, green peppers, salad greens	scurvy – bleeding gums, gingivitis, haemorrhages in skin, eyes, nose, weakness, muscle and joint pain	relatively nontoxic. May get gastrointestinal symptoms with doses higher than 3g daily
Vitamin A (Retinol Beta-carotene)	0.75 (2500 IU)	beta-carotene is widely distributed in green vegetables. Retinol is present in halibut liver oil, liver, milk, butter, cheese, margarine and eggs	scaly skin, night blindness, poor hair, eye ulceration, burning, itching eyes	headache, nausea and vomiting, dry itchy skin, loss of appetite, loss of hair
Vitamin D	0.01 (400 IU)	cod liver oil, eggs, dairy products, kippers, mackerel, salmon, tuna. Non-dietary source: sunlight	rickets (bone deformities) in children. Osteomalacia in adults	nausea and vomiting, diarrhoea, loss of weight, kidney damage
Vitamin E (Tocopherol)	30	cod liver oil, peanuts, seeds, green leafy vegetables, shrimps, olive oil, pulses	possibly anaemia, lethargy, decreased sexual interest, muscle weakness	relatively nontoxic
Vitamin K (Phyllo quinone)	0.03	green leafy vegetables, meats, liver and beans, fruits and meats	conditions associated with severe bleeding; internal haemorrhages in the newborn	relatively nontoxic. Synthetic forms at high doses may cause jaundice

*Usual diet provides 0.15-0.3   ** Usual diet provides 500-1000*

	Recommended Daily Intake (mg)	Best Dietary Sources	Effects of Deficiency	Effects of Excess

inerals

	Recommended Daily Intake (mg)	Best Dietary Sources	Effects of Deficiency	Effects of Excess
lcium	500-1000	milk, cheese, dark green vegetables, dried legumes	stunted growth, rickets in children, osteoporosis (weak, thin bones), tetany	not reported in man
osphorus	800-1000	milk, cheese, meat, poultry, grains	weakness, loss of appetite, bone pain, loss of calcium, irritability, pins and needles, tremors, confusion	can cause diarrhoea and calcification in soft tissues
phur	800	a constituent of all proteins: eggs, fish, meat, chicken, milk, cheese, pulses, wholegrains	related to protein deficiency	excess may lead to poor growth
tassium	2500	meats, milk, many fruits especially dried, molasses, raw vegetables, coffee, tea, chocolate	muscular weakness, paralysis, vomiting, loss of appetite, low blood pressure, intense thirst, confusion	muscular weakness, mental apathy, weakness of heart muscle, death
loride	2000	common salt	muscle cramps, mental apathy, reduced appetite. Occurs with sodium deficiency	vomiting
dium	2500	common salt	muscle cramps, mental apathy, reduced appetite	high blood pressure
gnesium	350	wholegrains, nuts, green leafy vegetables, shrimps, bananas	weakness, vertigo, hyperactivity in children, muscle cramps, palpitations	diarrhoea
n	10-18	eggs, lean meats, legumes, wholegrains, green leafy vegetables, shellfish	iron-deficiency anaemia (weakness, reduced resistance to infection)	excess usually excreted in faeces
orine	2	drinking water, tea, seafood	higher frequency of tooth decay	mottling of teeth, increased bone density, neurological disturbances
nc	15	widely distributed in foods	eczema, hair loss, mental apathy, post-natal depression, white spots on nails	very large doses may cause nausea, vomiting, diarrhoea
pper	2	meats, liver, drinking water	anaemia, brittle bones, poor hair, loss of sense of taste	low toxicity but can cause nausea, vomiting, diarrhoea
enium	0.2	seafood, meat, grains	anaemia (rare)	hair loss, abnormal nails, lassitude
nganese	5	widely distributed in foods: cereals, nuts, pulses, fruit, vegetables	associated with diabetes, disturbances of nervous system, heart disease	very rare but include lethargy, lack of control of voluntary movements, generalized disease of nervous system
line	0.14	sea fish and shellfish, many vegetables, fruit and cereals	goitre (enlarged thyroid), hypothyroidism – apathy, weight gain, coarse skin, drowsiness	very high intakes depress thyroid activity
olybdenum	0.5	legumes, cereals, organ meats, wholegrains	not reported in man	gout
romium	0.2	egg yolk, molasses, meat, hard cheese	nervous complaints, increased blood cholesterol, heart disease	none reported
balt	***	green leafy vegetables, fish	not reported in man	industrial exposure: dermatitis and diseases of red blood cells
ater	1.5 litres per day	solid foods, liquids, drinking water	thirst, dehydration	headaches, nausea, oedema, high blood pressure

Required as Vitamin B-12

Nutritional recommendations for a healthy diet

With the abundance of information gathered from the study of nutrition, and the research connecting diet with disease, what conclusions can we come to about what is a healthy, balanced diet?

The latest figures recommended by WHO refer to the proportion of nutrients as a percentage of the total calorie intake since the actual calorie needs of an individual vary with the amount of physical activity and work performed (see Table 14, pages 112–113).

The WHO Report recommends the following nutrient proportions of total calories:

* complex carbohydrates – 70–75%, consisting of wholegrain cereals, fruit, vegetables and pulses

* protein – 10–15% of calories, more from fish and poultry than red meat

* total fat – 15–30%, but not more than 10% as saturated (animal) fat

* sugar – less than 10%, ideally no added sugar at all

* dietary fibre – 25–35g per day which will be taken in automatically if 70% of the diet is in the form of complex carbohydrates as recommended

What does this mean in practical terms? What should your diet, ideally, consist of?

Daily

* plenty of wholemeal cereals: wholemeal bread, wholegrain rice and pasta, porridge oats

* plenty of all kinds of fruit and vegetables, including beans, lentils, potatoes (with skin wherever possible); more specifically, 1 lb fruit and vegetables consisting of one portion green leafy vegetable, one portion yellow vegetable, one mixed salad, two portions fruit or berries

* plenty of fish; all kinds (including shellfish occasionally) grilled, steamed or poached

* poultry and game; without skin, roasted, grilled, poached or steamed

* skimmed milk, low-fat cheeses

* limited amounts of vegetable oils and margarine high in polyunsaturates

* water, as much as you like (bottled preferably)

Occasionally

* red meat, liver, kidneys, bacon, ham; lean, not more than three times a week

* eggs, three egg yolks only per week

* cheese: camembert, brie, parmesan, mozzarella, Dutch cheeses

* ice cream, sorbet, low-fat yoghurt

* all kinds of nuts

* alcohol: beer, wine

Avoid if possible

* processed foods, fried foods, fatty meat, sausages, meat pies, salted/smoked/cured foods, cakes, pastry, puddings, biscuits, sweets, toffee, chocolate, jam

These recommendations are a far cry from the 'meat and two veg.' on which most of us were raised. It will be interesting to see how shops and restaurants respond to the possible forthcoming revolution in public taste and the ensuing demand for simpler, more wholesome foods – a diet that will possibly be a lot cheaper too.

Alcohol

Food needs lots of liquid to wash it down. For a long time, before tea, coffee and chocolate became popular beverages, in the seventeenth century the fluids to drink with meals apart from water, which was often undrinkable, were alcoholic grain-based beers, ales, mead and, in countries where grapes grew, wine.

Fermented drinks have been known to exist for thousands of years but distilling was only discovered in the first century AD. Eventually, refinement of the method of distilling wine resulted, in the twelfth century, in almost pure alcohol – a liquid known as *aqua vita* (water of life) or 'brandy'. Four centuries later, spirits were being distilled from fermented grains in the form of gin, schnapps, akvavit and, in Ireland and Scotland, whisky.

Besides being a thirst-quencher, alcohol has become a cornerstone of any, and almost all, social occasions and an utterly normal portion of many people's daily diet. What is often not realized is the power of alcohol to destroy and the care with which it needs to be regarded.

In moderate quantities, there is reason to believe that alcohol may contribute to health. One study that mentioned HDL cholesterol levels before and after drinking half a bottle of red wine a day for six weeks, suggested that this level of alcohol intake would protect against coronary heart disease and gall stones. Another study carried out mental tests on elderly men and suggested that alcohol sharpened their wits.

Moderate to heavy consumption of alcohol may be associated with increased blood pressure which, in turn, increases the risk of coronary heart disease and stroke. Drinking more than 42 alcohol units a week has been linked with a four-fold increase of strokes in middle-aged men. However, epidemiological studies have consistently shown that *moderate* alcohol consumption protects against coronary heart disease. Recently, a study carried out on a large population in New Zealand went one step further. It showed that men who had had a heart attack and men who had died of coronary heart disease were more likely never to have been drinkers. Furthermore, drinking up to 56 units of alcohol a week was found to be associated with a significantly reduced risk of both heart attacks and fatal CHD in both men *and* women: the reduced risk was, in general, even greater in women than in men. This study also showed that *non-smokers* who drank up to this amount benefited even more from the protective association between alcohol and CHD.

Whilst this is good news for those of us who enjoy wine with meals or a pint or two at the pub, *excess* alcohol consumption is associated with damage to the other parts of the body. It is important that alcohol consumption is kept within moderate limits when one considers that alcohol has been estimated to lead to 28,000 deaths annually in England and Wales,

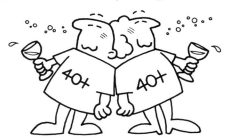

and the cost of treating alcohol-related illnesses in Britain was calculated at £167 million in 1986.

Heavy drinking is causally related to cancers of the liver, mouth, pharynx, oesophagus and larynx, the hypothesis being that drinkers suffer from certain nutrient deficiencies that may increase the susceptibility of the lining cells of the mouth, throat and oesophagus to becoming cancerous. A link has also been found between excess alcohol and cancer of the rectum, and, in women, cancer of the breast.

How often have you heard someone of a certain age say – or indeed have remarked yourself – 'I cannot drink like I used to when I was younger. It knocks me out; I feel too tired to work; I cannot function well.'

The explanation of this creeping incapacity lies in the fact that alcohol consumption in middle or older age has a greater effect on the liver and the brain than when younger. The liver, along with other organs, shrinks with age so its capacity to handle alcohol diminishes. Cirrhosis of the liver is the major chronic disease caused by excess alcohol. When the capacity of the liver to detoxify alcohol is overloaded, liver cells are destroyed and replaced with scar tissue. There is evidence that women are more susceptible to the development of cirrhosis as a result of alcohol than men.

The effect of alcohol on the brain, whether one's own or another's, is, no doubt, recognizable if not familiar. The long-term chronic effect of excess alcohol may be brain damage. It takes about ten years of heavy drinking to produce this damage: ageing processes may be accelerated and interfere with reasoning capacity and normal ability to problem-solve in everyday life.

Alcohol may also cause overweight as it contains a large number of calories (7 Kcal per gram).

Pregnant women who drink may produce the 'foetal alcohol syndrome' in their offspring that involves mental and general growth retardation. The full-blown form of the syndrome may occur in children of women who drink more than eight alcoholic drinks (units) per day. Other effects, such as low birth weight and an increased risk of still-birth, occur at a much more *moderate* alcohol intake – two units or more (20g alcohol) per day. The startling fact is that alcohol is one of the commonest causes of birth abnormalities in developed countries. Drinking when breast feeding is also inadvisable as alcohol can be passed to the baby through breast milk.

Notwithstanding the increased protection women who enjoy a drink appear to have with respect to CHD, women are particularly susceptible to alcohol, partly because they are generally smaller than men and partly because they have more fat and less water in their bodies. When women drink, the alcohol is not diluted to the same extent and stays in the body longer. This effect of increased alcohol concentration is particularly true just before a menstrual period or just before ovulation. Also, alcohol is absorbed more slowly into the bloodstream and remains in the body longer in individuals who are on the pill.

Finally, alcohol is a major cause of accidents. Almost half of all road accidents in this and other developed countries have alcohol as

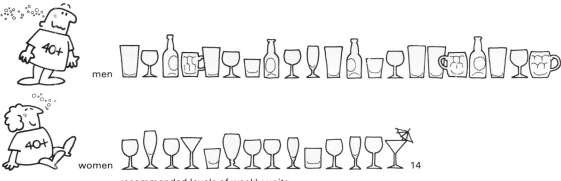

men 21

women 14

recommended levels of weekly units

a causal factor; it also contributes significantly to drownings and boating accidents.

But, as an oenophile myself, I am the first to ask, 'What can I drink without damaging myself or others?' The current recommendations are as follows:

* In men – up to 21 units* per week

* In women – up to 14 units* per week

If possible, two or three days a week should be alcohol-free.

Are you alcohol dependent?

Try this 'CAGE' questionnaire, devised for detecting alcoholism by Dr J. A. Ewing:

> Have you ever felt you should cut down on your drinking?
> Have other people annoyed you by criticizing your drinking?
> Have you ever felt guilty about drinking?
> Have you ever taken a drink in the morning (an eye-opener) to steady your nerves or to get rid of a hangover?

A 'Yes' to two or more questions indicates you

*1 unit = half a pint of beer = 1 glass of wine = 1 glass of sherry = 1 single (pub measure) spirits = a measure of vermouth or aperitif.

may be at risk of alcohol dependence and may need to seek guidance and help.

There is a difference between problem drinking and alcohol dependence. Alcohol dependence, scientists now agree, is the result of genetic predisposition towards a craving for alcohol. As a result of this discovery, alcoholism has come to be regarded as a disease. Problem drinking, on the other hand, may occur from habitual, persistent heavy drinking as a response to long-term stress; it can bring about bodily changes leading to craving but the triggering factor is environmental or social rather than genetic.

The gene in question, referred to as the alcogene, may also be associated with other kinds of addiction. It is estimated that about 10% of the population may be affected; this figure was arrived at from studies of Vietnam War veterans who became addicted to drugs whilst serving in Vietnam. With rehabilitation, all but 10% recovered. It was concluded that the remaining 10% were physiologically addicted due to an inherent predisposition, i.e., a genetic factor.

Problem drinking can be avoided by being aware of the social, psychological and environmental stresses that may contribute towards it. But for the individual with the alcogene, drinking alcohol can produce the effects of a physical 'allergy' combined with a mental compulsion. These individuals are better off never touching a drop.

SIX

Weight – how to control it

In France, Babar the Elephant has been chosen to represent to children the image of good healthy eating. Babar might at first seem an odd choice for this job, as elephants are not renowned for having a svelte appearance. But, perhaps that is the whole point. The French have cleverly attempted to disentangle the business of eating healthily from a present-day unhealthy preoccupation with thinness. This cultural obsession with acquiring a reed-like body shape used to be an 'adults only' fixation. But today girls as young as eight years of age have caught it and deprive themselves of food to avoid getting fat.

Babar is wise and wonderful, a truly reliable soul who knows what to do for the best. In Elephantland, there is no such thing as a fat elephant or a thin elephant; Babar, Celeste and all the other elephants are simply elephant-sized. Like all healthy animals, they eat what is right for them. Choosing Babar as the mascot for good healthy eating could be a stroke of genius.

Meanwhile, back at home, the slimming business is booming; the sale of low-calorie meals and drinks produces £6m a week – a 20% increase on last year. According to the Office of Population Censuses and Surveys, in 1990 almost half the male population and a third of women, that is nearly 21 million or 40% of adults, were overweight; the figures have been rising steadily in the last decade.

Why does body weight increase with age? The average American gains a pound per year from the age of twenty-five onwards; by age forty-five, he or she may have a total weight gain of 20 pounds, but a *fat* weight gain of 30 pounds! This extra 10 pounds of fat is accounted for by the gradual loss, with age, of lean body weight, mainly muscle and bone, at the rate of half a pound a year. Reduced lean body weight means less calories in food are needed. But, if food intake remains unchanged, more food than required is ingested, fat accumulates and body weight goes up. This 'creeping obesity' is helped along by diminishing levels of physical activity.

Half the women in this country claim to be on a reducing diet and most of them abandoned their last diet without success. Whilst two-thirds of the world starves, the rest is slimming.

Why are some people fatter than others?

Greed and gluttony have always been blamed for excess weight. Self-righteous moralists have been known to condemn with unrepentant harshness the visibly well fed for manifestly indulging in a deadly sin. Stout people are an easy target at which to aim disapproval as they can hardly hide their bulk. Whilst over-eating certainly results in weight gain, the reality is more complex.

The genetic footprint makes its stamp

Tweedledum and Tweedledee would have looked the same even if they had been separated in infancy and brought up in completely different families. It may be said without fear of contradiction that Mr and Mrs Tweedle were almost certainly similarly rotund. There is an 88% chance of inheriting obesity from

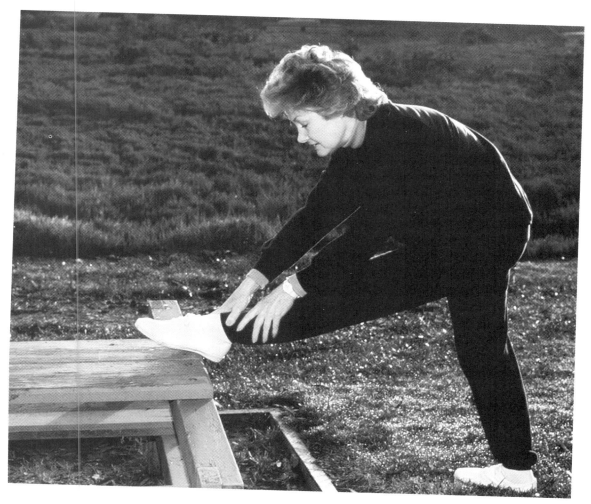

Exercise helps control weight

parents. The implication is that a genetic defect may account for excessive appetite in obese people. In addition, errors in the genetic code, determining the production of a number of key enzymes, cause increased accumulation of fat and also a diminished rate of usage of fat from the stores. This research paints a picture of obesity that is a long way from the simple concept of over-eating. This doesn't mean that people from fat families cannot control their weight. But it takes extra care and concentration if they are to avoid excessive weight-gain.

Inactivity

Reduced energy expenditure has been studied in relation to the development of obesity. Infants who become overweight by one year of age were found to have been considerably less active than normal-weight babies at three months. A number of studies have shown that obese children tend to participate less in physical activities than those with normal body weight. Other studies do not support these findings. So, the question of inactivity in the development of obesity remains open.

Fat cells – how many/how large?

The number of fat cells in an adult remains constant, the number having been determined by a gradual increase in fat cells during childhood and the growth spurt of early adolescence.

When excess food is stored as fat, the fat cells literally swell up like fat-filled balloons; when a diet is restricted and stored fat is used as energy, fat cells give up their fat and shrink. Weight-loss in adults who are not grossly obese is due purely to shrinkage in the size of fat cells; there is no change in the number of these cells. When normal food habits are abandoned, like at Christmas or on holidays when more food is eaten than necessary, the shrunken fat cells fill up again and those stubborn extra rolls appear.

Comparisons of the number of fat cells in naturally slim people compared to fat people show an enormous variation. For example, a non-obese person has approximately 25–30 billion fat cells, a person classified as obese may have 75 billion, whereas the number of fat cells in the 'extremely obese' may be as high as 260 billion! The 'extremely obese' individual is one who is nearly twice the normal weight and shoots off the end of the over-weight graph. No more fat can be squeezed into this individual's existing fat cells, so more cells are recruited from an immature cell pool to increase the cell number. This only occurs in these cases of massive obesity.

How is weight controlled?

Each person's body seems to have a genetically preferred volume of fat cells; any changes above or below this level trigger a complex chain of events affecting the basal metabolic rate (BMR), the aim of which is to preserve a constant body weight. If calories are restricted and weight is lost, the body, apparently anticipating a crisis of famine, war and pestilence, responds by reducing its metabolic rate so that it runs at a lower energy cost and can exist on less food.

This self-regulating mechanism conserves fat that would otherwise be used as fuel, so the fat-cell volume is preserved. Equally, if you eat more to try to raise your body weight, your metabolic rate will speed up to try to keep your weight stable. This concept of the body 'guarding' a preferred weight is the basis of the 'set point' theory of weight maintenance. It is simply an expression of the body's adaptive efforts to protect its stores of energy; the more these stores are 'stolen', the more the body defends them against further attacks.

You may also notice when dieting that you have less desire to move about or involve yourself in physical activity. This inertia is another attempt by the body to defend its weight by using less energy. It is a combination of these quite remarkable mechanisms that control an individual's body weight over the years within a relatively small range. Obviously, food intake, and therefore the amount of energy available in calories, varies from day to day and yet body weight remains remarkably constant. If these mechanisms did

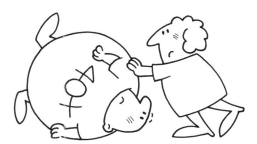

not operate, eating just one extra potato chip a day (10 Kcal per day) would result in a weight gain of approximately 1 lb per year (10 Kcal × 365 days per year = 3650 Kcal per year = 1 lb fat). But, of course, this does not happen. The body is able to adjust in order to maintain a set point of weight.

The set point is not writ in stone, however. There is evidence that it can be adjusted. One factor that seems to adjust the set point downwards is exercise. An increased level of exercise causes an increase in metabolic rate and, contrary to popular belief, a decrease in appetite and calorie intake. This appetite-depressant effect of exercise is thought to be due to a chemical substance produced for 60–90 minutes after vigorous physical activity, together with increased levels of stress hormones, increased body temperature and reduced insulin, all of which suppress appetite. Less food intake, together with a higher metabolic rate, will result in a drop in body weight to a new 'preferred' weight.

When this new lower weight is reached, further increases in exercise levels are matched with increases in calorie intake; in effect, the body has reached a new 'set point' and begins to guard the new weight against further raids on its energy stores. It is not known exactly how this fascinating mechanism works except that exercise training brings into play a number of otherwise little-used systems that are energy-expensive to maintain, rather like a car that, when driven more than usual, will require more servicing, more petrol and more oil.

It seems that the energy for these exercise-related activities is preferentially obtained from stored fat (and not from lean body tissue) because exercise has a specific, fat-mobilizing effect. In females, though, the original 'set point' is guarded much more vigorously and it is harder for women to establish a lower 'set point'.

Risks associated with excess weight

The health consequences of obesity are numerous; they include: high blood pressure which is causally related to obesity and predisposes to strokes, heart disease and kidney disease; high blood cholesterol with a blood-fat profile characteristic of individuals at risk for CHD; diabetes of mature onset with associated heart disease, peripheral vascular disease, gangrene and kidney conditions; gall stones and several forms of cancer. In addition, excessive weight can interfere with respiratory function in chronic obstructive lung disease, and exacerbates pain in the hips, spine and knees in osteoarthritis.

Weight reduction is one of the most effective ways to lower blood pressure; it will also tend to normalize the blood-fat levels and the pain of arthritis will be relieved.

The Framingham study, named after a town in the USA in which the population was studied for twenty-six years to assess the incidence of heart disease, showed that obesity is a risk factor in its own right in CHD. The fatter you are the greater the risk, but there are health risks associated with being overweight even when not obese. It appears that where you 'wear' your fat can affect your health.

Are you an 'apple' or a 'pear'?

'Apples' like Humpty Dumpty distribute their fat around their middles, tending to build their round shape from the inside out and storing most of their abdominal fat within the abdominal cavity. 'Pears', on the other hand, distribute fat around the hips and thighs where it is stored just below the skin in the subcutaneous layer. Apples have an advantage in having very active enzymes that can create a rapid turnover and movement of 'gut' fat. So, apples who exercise are able to move their fat with relative ease. In pears, however, the fat cells in the hip and thigh regions are more stubborn and don't give up their fat so easily. Only during breast feeding are they willing to relinquish their greedily guarded fat stores. Since 'pears' are usually female, this suggests that hip and thigh fat stores represent an insurance so that when a woman has a baby she will have adequate energy supplies for nursing.

Being an 'apple' isn't all a bed of roses however. The fact that fat around the gut is more easily mobilized also means that a greater amount of mobilized fat is dumped into the blood stream. During exercise, this is a good

---

HOW TO TELL IF YOU'RE AN 'APPLE' OR A 'PEAR'

Find your waist: hip ratio

1. Measure your waist – don't breathe in!

2. Measure your hips

3. Divide waist measurement by hip measurement for waist:hip ratio

4. Ratios of less than 1.0 for men and 0.8 for women are fine. If your waist:hip ratio is greater than either of these, you need to lose some weight

   For example

   For a woman: if your waist is 28ins and hips are 38ins, waist:hip ratio is 0.74

   For a man: if your waist is 34ins and hips are 38ins, waist:hip ratio is 0.9

---

thing because the fat is available as fuel for working muscles. But if stress has caused this release of fat into the blood, and no exercise is taken to use it up as fuel, it is made into cholesterol which is deposited in the walls of arteries causing narrowing and predisposing to atherosclerosis. Consequently, 'apples', whether men or women, have a higher risk of coronary heart disease, due to higher blood cholesterol levels that result from the easier mobilization of abdominal fat.

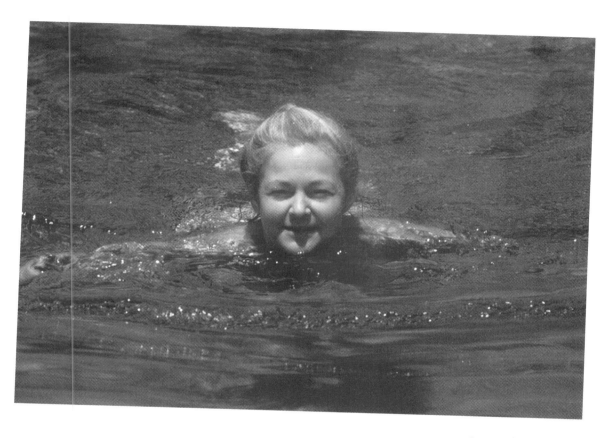

How fat are you?

Swimming can be as gentle or strenuous as you care to make it

Obesity and overweight are not necessarily the same thing. An athlete may be overweight compared with the average for his or her height but the extra weight may be due to a large frame or extra muscle development, rather than excess fat. Such an athlete weighs more than the average but he is not obese. Obesity on the other hand refers to an excess of body fat. In general, obesity and body weight do go hand-in-hand; the greater the body weight the greater the amount of body fat. But, weight alone is not a satisfactory in-dicator of excess body fat, neither does it give any idea of the composition of the various major structural components of the human body – muscle, fat and bone. Traditionally, standard age-height-weight tables have been used to assess an individual's degree of excess weight, but they reveal little about a person's body composition which, as in the case of the athlete cited above, can vary considerably at any given height and weight.

Essential and storage fat

Essential fat is stored in the bone marrow, heart, lungs, liver, spleen, kidneys, intestines, muscles, orbit and central nervous system; in women, additional essential fat depots are situated in the breasts and the pelvis. This kind of fat, as its name implies, is necessary for normal body functions. *Storage fat* is a nutritional reserve and accumulates in fat depots under the skin surface and around the internal organs where it acts as a cushion to protect from trauma. The proportional distribution of storage fat in men and women is similar – 12% in males, 15% in females. But there is a marked sex difference in essential fat which, in women, averages 12% compared with 3% in men. This four-fold higher amount in women is probably related to child-bearing and other hormone-related functions. It appears that an individual cannot reduce his or her body fat below the essential fat level and still maintain good health.

Body Mass Index

Body Mass Index (BMI) is being used more and more to assess body composition and classify obesity. It gives a more accurate estimate of obesity than the old standard age-height-weight tables.

To find your BMI, divide your weight (in kilos) by your height (in metres) squared. For example, say you are 1.80 metres tall and weigh 71.3 kg.

$$\text{BMI} = \frac{\text{Weight}}{\text{Height}^2} = \frac{71.3}{1.80^2} = \frac{71.3}{3.24} = 22$$

A healthy BMI range is approximately 20–25; less than 20 is underweight. If your BMI is between 25–30, you are overweight; weight loss is recommended as your health could suffer. If your BMI is 30–40, you are obese; weight loss should be considered a priority. A BMI of more than 40 indicates that health is seriously at risk (see Table 8).

Losing weight

The energy balance equation

Fat accumulates and body weight increases if the total calories ingested as food exceed the daily energy requirements. The energy balance equation states:

When food in = energy output, body weight is stable
When food in is greater than energy output, body weight increases
When food in is less than energy output, body weight decreases

The energy balance equation can be affected by:

1. 'Energy input', i.e. calories as food, reduced to below energy output

2. Increased 'energy output', i.e. physical activity

3. Reduced food intake *and* increased physical activity

We will now consider each of these methods of weight-loss in turn.

Table 8 **What is your Body Mass Index?**

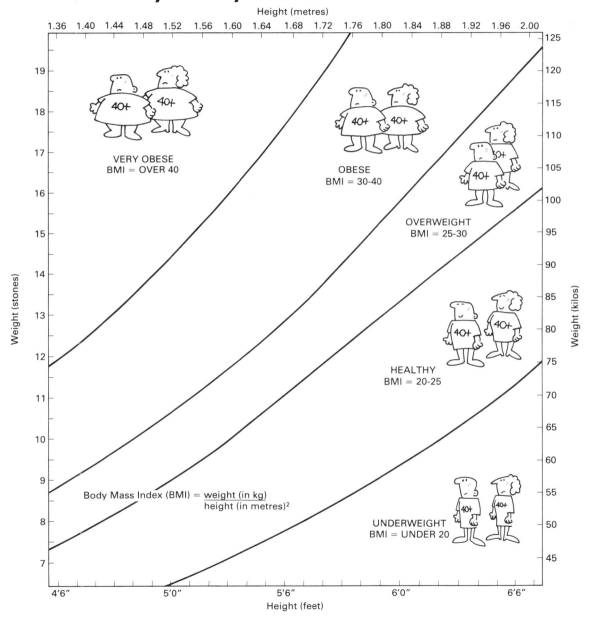

Weight-loss by dieting

FADS AND FALLACIES

Public susceptibility to fad diets with their 'quick-fix' promises of rapid weight-loss seems infinite. Magazines emblazoned with 'Lose 5 lbs in a weekend!' or 'Drop 7 lbs in 7 days' on their covers sell more copies. People, it seems, are more than willing to abandon their innate logic and buy into the latest magic spell. But the reason that magazines and newspapers can go on recycling the same fallacious claims is that they don't work. If they did, people who tried them would lose their excess weight and would have no more use for reducing diets or the magazines promoting them. It is certainly the case that several pounds can be lost in a few days with severe calorie restriction. But most of it is water that is replaced as soon as normal eating is resumed.

Similarly, with low carbohydrate/low calorie diets, the body's water is severely depleted along with glucose and glycogen stores in the liver and muscles. Ketosis occurs (loss of appetite, ammonia smell on breath, increased flow of urine) as fat from depots is metabolized for energy, which causes a further water loss – as much as 3–5 lbs a week. But, as soon as a normal diet is resumed, carbohydrate stores are replenished and water is replaced. So, body weight increases by 4–5 lbs during the first one or two days after stopping the diet.

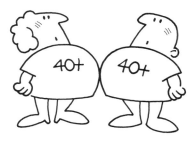

'YO-YO' DIETING

Quick weight-loss with severe dietary restriction is appealing and can be achieved with, for instance, semi-starvation diets like the VLCDs (Very Low Calorie Diet) in obese people under medical supervision. But, regardless of how successful a particular weight-loss method may be, most people gain the weight back. People in the public eye, such as Oprah Winfrey and Luciano Pavarotti, have the disadvantage of riding this weight-loss/gain roller coaster in full view whilst demonstrating the extreme difficulties many people encounter in trying to keep their body weight down. Repeated cycles of weight-loss and weight-gain are known as 'yo-yo' dieting. With each failed attempt at dieting, losing weight becomes more difficult and weight-gain more rapid because a number of changes appear to come into play in the body that are counterproductive to weight-loss. These are as follows:

1. The metabolic rate drops following a period of underfeeding in an effort to conserve fat stores in response to what the body 'perceives' as starvation (see 'set point' theory above). This lowering of the body's energy

requirements, perhaps by as much as 30%, is thought to be a key factor in the oft-repeated failure of many dieters to reach and maintain a target weight. When normal eating is resumed, the metabolic rate goes up again but probably not as high as it was to begin with. During the dieting period, the body is adapting to energy restriction by using less energy to function. It improves its fuel efficiency. Subsequent attempts at weight-loss are somewhat thwarted by this improved efficiency. So, losing weight becomes progressively more difficult.

2. When body weight is lost, lean tissue is lost as well as fat – mainly water and protein, especially muscle. When weight is regained, the lost muscle tends to be replaced with fat. So, you end up with more fat than you started with before dieting. This decrease in lean body mass, combined with the age-related decrease mentioned in Chapter 3, contributes significantly to a further drop in metabolic rate.

3. When dieting, people frequently feel lethargic and consequently tend to move around much less and use up less energy in physical activity.

4. Appetite is lost during dieting due to the accumulation of ketones as body fat is 'burned' for energy. But the appetite returns with a vengeance when dieting stops. Excess food is eaten and is converted to body fat.

5. It may be more difficult to stick to a maintenance diet after a period of weight-loss dieting because a taste for high calorie foods develops.

The repeated weight fluctuation characteristic of 'yo-yo' dieting carries its own health risks, in particular an increased risk of heart disease because the regained weight tends to accumulate in the belly, in the 'apple' area of distribution. Weight cycling may also increase an individual's risk of developing gall bladder disease, especially gall stone formation.

Psychologically, repeated failure to maintain weight-loss can strike a blow to self-esteem and may lead to eating disorders such as bingeing and bulimia nervosa. A study of 368 high-school and sixty-three college wrestlers in the USA demonstrated this problem. The wrestlers subjected themselves to severe food restriction to make the weight in their event prior to competition, a process associated with a great deal of anxiety. After the matches, many of the wrestlers described feeling out of control when eating.

In 1990, to avoid these hazardous and traumatic attempts at weight-loss, the US Departments of Agriculture and of Health and Human Services issued new guidelines recommending that people reduce weight at a safe rate of ½–1 lb per week (the previous recommendation had been a weekly loss of 1–2 lbs). One pound of fat contains 3500 kilo calories, so to lose 1 lb per week, you must reduce your food intake by 500 calories per day below your normal daily weight-maintaining level. But only about 70% of the weight lost by cutting calories is fat, the rest is muscle.

Weight-loss by exercising

Exercise alone can result in weight-loss by burning more calories than you eat but it tends to be a rather slow process. A good distance runner completing a 26-mile marathon in 2½ hours at a pace of about 10 mph uses up less than a pound of body fat as fuel. The total energy cost of a marathon tends to be the same regardless of pace, oddly enough. However, regular physical training involving moderate to vigorous exercise, such as running, jogging, cycling, swimming, rowing, dancing, vigorous sports or games, for 20–30 minutes each session, or brisk walking for 45–60 minutes, three or more days per week, results in significant changes in body composition. There is an increase in lean (fat-free) body weight due to increased muscle mass, and a decrease in body fat. Body weight may not change in the early stages of such a programme.

The most important factor to consider when exercising to achieve weight-loss is the total energy cost of the exercise. If 300–500 Kcal per session are used, an individual can lose 1 lb of fat in 7–12 exercise sessions if food

Jogging can be moderate or vigorous exercise

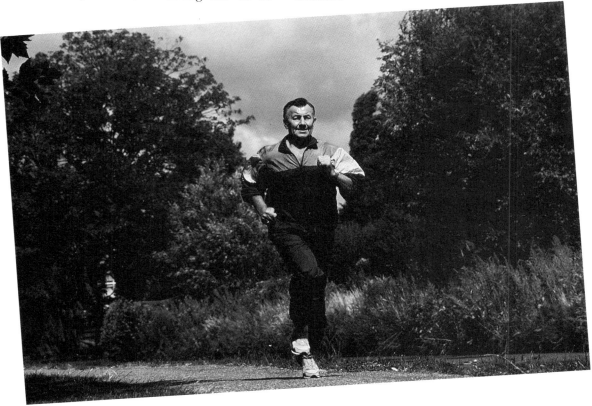

intake remains constant.

If you were to jog at a moderate rate for thirty minutes, four times a week, you could lose 4 lbs of fat in three months. Since your body shape would be changing as more muscle developed and fat was lost, changes in your body would be more noticeable than the figures suggest. If you walked briskly for an hour a day, every day, you could lose 1 lb of fat each week, and 12 lbs in three months, assuming that your food intake remained the same. The use of body fat as fuel is helped by the specific fat-mobilizing effect of exercise.

In addition to the basic energy cost of the exercise when it is being performed, the metabolic rate of the body when it is *resting* is also enhanced. This post-exercise 'afterburn' effect was found to be of a greater magnitude and duration with high-intensity exercise. The burning of extra calories even when resting means that this kind of exercise is particularly helpful in promoting weight-loss. However, low-intensity exercise performed for longer produces weight-loss benefits similar to those of high-intensity exercise of shorter duration (hence the marathon statement above).

For people caught in the 'yo-yo' dieting trap, whose metabolism has slid into low gear, exercise can be the most effective stimulant to get their metabolism back into high gear again. Also, whereas weight-loss by diet alone causes a significant loss of muscle mass (up to 36% in one study), exercise appears to protect against this loss so that almost all the lost body weight is fat. The addition of muscle strengthening exercises, like weight training or machine weights, is effective in helping to maintain or increase the lean body mass.

Weight-loss by dieting and exercising

A number of studies have shown that the most effective and the safest way to lose excess weight is with a combination of diet and exercise. In addition to the beneficial effects on lean body mass of exercise alone, fat is lost at a faster rate and to a greater degree than with either diet only or exercise only. A modest reduction of kilo calories, say 250 per day, combined with an increase in physical activity to account for a further 250 kilo calories a day will result in a loss of 1 lb of fat per week. This could be managed by cutting out one dessert and walking three miles in forty-five minutes each day. Fortunately, the calorie-using effects of exercise are cumulative; if a little exercise is performed regularly, the effect over a period of time can be dramatic.

Sticking to a restricted diet may be easier with a diet-plus-exercise regime because of the appetite-suppressant effect of exercise. Also, the sense of well-being, diminished anxiety and improved self-esteem, described by people who exercise, can help you to adhere to the diet/exercise programme in the long term.

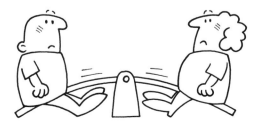

SEVEN

Stress

What is stress?

Stress is often viewed as a modern-day scourge. We talk of stress-related symptoms of disease, of the stresses and strains of everyday living and of stress in the work-place. But, we, of the twentieth century, cannot claim to have discovered stress. In the seventeenth century, it stood for hardship, straits, adversity and affliction and was regarded as a kind of uncontrollable monster that could rear its ugly head and fell an individual at a stroke. The word 'stress' was derived from 'distress', and the two became synonymous. Stress was definitely something to be avoided; it was seen as a destructive force which, if allowed to exert itself, could demolish the best-laid plans and cause damage and breakdown.

At about the same time, John Locke, the English physician and philosopher, was laying the foundations of physiology with his theories and notions relating life experiences and emotions to hormonal and biochemical changes in the body. Locke realized that stress did not simply refer to irksome external forces or strokes of fate visited on a hapless victim, but that it denoted a physiological response, the level of which depended on an individual's nature and constitution: 'Though the faculties of the mind are improved by exercise, yet they must not be put to a stress beyond their strength.'

A century and a half later in France, whilst Louis Pasteur was propounding the Germ Theory of Disease, Claude Bernard, a French physiologist, was asking the question: Why doesn't everyone become infected with 'germs' or bacteria in an epidemic? Why do some people remain healthy whilst others succumb to the infection? Bernard suggested that it was the internal environment (*milieu intérieur*) of a living creature that was the key to the maintenance of health or the development of disease, and that to be healthy the organism must keep this internal state as constant as possible despite changes in the external environment or challenges from bacteria and other infectious micro-organisms. From Bernard's work on the *milieu intérieur* the general concept of resistance to disease emerged.

Scientists began to identify how the body reacts to stressful events and situations. It was becoming clear that stress did not simply refer to unpleasant, damaging or toxic factors in the external environment that act on the individual. Stress also encompasses the reactions of the body to strains placed upon it.

This notion that the body is constantly attempting to return to a balanced internal state or stable norm in the face of constantly changing and challenging environmental conditions was later referred to as *homeostasis* by Walter B. Cannon, an eminent American physiologist of the 1930s.

From this response-based view of stress the idea emerged that, though the word stress has negative connotations and is often associated with deleterious and damaging effects, it is not necessarily always bad, unpleasant or 'distressing'. Stress is also not something to be avoided. Indeed, since stressors are encountered constantly by all living organisms including plants, it is not something that can be avoided. In a real sense, if you are alive you are under some degree of stress. An amoeba,

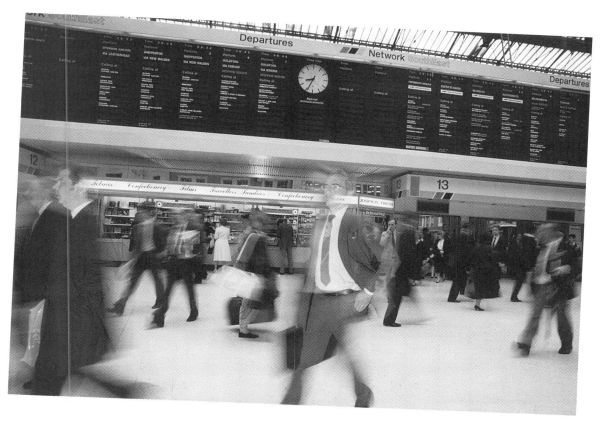

Commuting – a very stressful activity!

as it reacts to stimuli by moving away or putting out pseudopodia to engulf a foreign body, is a good example of a simple unicellular organism coping with stressors by adjusting and protecting itself in order to survive.

Similarly, human beings are constantly adapting to sources of stress in their environment but in a way that involves a highly complex response pattern. Moreover, stress is necessary to achieve results; motivation, development, growth and change are all associated with a degree of stress. Problems arise when the levels of stress become excessive and unmanageable.

In the 1950s, Professor Hans Selye, the acknowledged founder of the scientific approach to stress, started to throw a more analytical light on the subject. He had spent many years in the laboratory researching at a cellular level the biochemical mechanisms of adaptation to the stress of life. He concluded that, notwithstanding the multiplicity of manifestations of stress – pain, fear, excitement, exhaustion, grief, anxiety, agitation, withdrawal, etc. – experienced as a result of any number of unique life events or stressors, the biochemical changes in the human body were essentially the same and were the characteristic responses for coping with *any* type of demand. According to Selye, 'it is immaterial whether the agent or situation we face is pleasant or unpleasant', or that the emotions felt are agreeable or uncomfortable. All that matters is that an urgent demand is being made on the body to adapt or readjust. The excitement of a marriage can be just as stressful to the bride

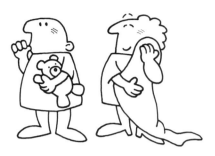

and groom as the grief felt at the death of a spouse even though the emotions experienced are totally different. But Selye asserted that, in both situations, the biochemical reactions in the people concerned were identical.

Selye called this non-specific response to stress the General Adaptation Syndrome (GAS); he identified three stages: (1) the alarm reaction; (2) the stage of resistance; and (3) the stage of exhaustion (see Figure 5). Selye likened these three stages to the major three stages of a human being's life: 'childhood (with its characteristic low resistance and excessive responses to any kind of stimulus), adulthood (during which adaptation to most commonly encountered agents has occurred and resistance is increased) and, finally, senility (characterized by irreversible loss of adaptability and eventual exhaustion) ending with death'.

Fight or flight

The initial 'alarm' stage evokes a response known as 'fight or flight'. As the name implies, the individual reacts to a signal he or she perceives as threatening, frightening or simply stimulating, by becoming alert,

aroused and prepared, physiologically, for action. Stress hormones, adrenalin and noradrenalin (known as catecholamines), secreted by the middle part of the adrenal glands and by the sympathetic nervous system, cause a number of immediate adjustments in the body's systems that prepare the individual for an acute emergency; heart rate and blood pressure rise; blood flow is directed away from the skin and internal organs towards the brain and muscle where it is most urgently needed; muscle tension increases; breathing tubes in the lungs expand to allow a greater intake of air; pupils in the eyes enlarge to allow more light to enter; glucose normally stored in the liver pours into the blood to provide a source of readily available energy for physical activity, and fat is mobilized from fat depots into the blood stream as a back-up source of energy.

The proportion of adrenalin to noradrenalin varies with the emotion experienced: fear produces a preponderance of adrenalin whilst noradrenalin is more typical of aggression. These two hormones appear instantly and are the first line of defence in stress. But, though they appear promptly on the scene they cannot sustain resistance as their effects are fairly short-lived. The second line of defence occurs a few minutes later when the adrenocorticotrophic hormone (ACTH – a hormone which is essential to survival and the body's ability to cope with stress), from the pituitary gland in the brain, stimulates the secretion of corticoid hormones from the adrenal glands.

Cortisol, the most active steroid in the group, enables more prolonged adaptation to stress by creating readily available sources of

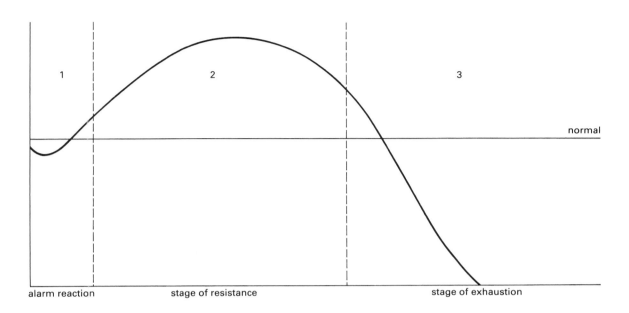

Figure 5 The three stages of reaction to stress (Selye's General Adaptation Syndrome)

energy by raising blood sugar from glycogen stores in the liver and mobilizing fat from depots, and metabolizing protein so that it can be used to repair damaged tissue. Cortisol also has an anti-inflammatory effect, preventing excess inflammation and scar tissue formation.

The body is literally prepared for battle or to beat a hasty retreat. This response is a survival mechanism that evolved to allow animals and humans to flee from predators and to hunt for food. Animals, even the domestic kind, still demonstrate the fight or flight response. Although your pet cat no longer needs to hunt to survive, it will still stalk and kill mice, voles and birds, and spit with rage, its hair standing on end.

The animal instinct to fight or flee still exists in human beings who show the same primitive patterns of physiological and biochemical arousal when confronted with situations perceived as dangerous and threatening; but, unlike animals, owing to our largely sedentary and 'civilized' way of life, we do not follow it through with physical activity and the release of aggression. In normal circumstances, the fight or flight response is no longer useful to contemporary Man.

Having a body primed for action but without any action taking place to utilize the surfeit of hormones and chemicals circulating in readiness for vigorous action, is detrimental to health. If this response is elicited often and to a sufficiently high level, stress-related symptoms may appear such as raised blood pressure; fat mobilized as an energy source is converted to cholesterol and laid down in the walls of arteries, causing the vessels to become narrower, the end result of which may well be coronary heart disease and a possibly fatal heart attack. Referring to the causes of heart disease, Dr Malcolm Carruthers, a stress specialist, says, 'It's not what you eat but what's eating you.'

Stress and exhaustion

When stress is intense, the three stages of GAS happen in quick succession and, with rest, the process is more or less reversible. But, inevitably, with each successive period or episode of stress, a cost is incurred in terms of 'wear and tear' on the organism. Selye made a connection between the gradual decline of the body and prolonged stress and ageing. He claimed that 'each period of stress, especially if it results from frustrating, unsuccessful struggles, leaves some irreversible chemical scars which accumulate to constitute the signs of tissue ageing'.

Adaptation to stress

The second stage of resistance to stress occurs if the stressor does not go away but the organism is able to adapt and re-establish a different level of function. Under the influence of stressors – like overwork, unemployment, marital discord, overcrowding, discrimination, noise, financial uncertainty, poor conditions at work, extremes of climate, commuting, difficult relationships, job insecurity, moving house, holidays, lack of sleep, family responsibilities, and many more – constant demands

are being made on the body to adapt and establish equilibrium. But the outcome appears to be a relentless chipping away and draining of the body's *capacity* to adapt to changing circumstances.

According to Selye's hypothesis, the body only has a finite amount of adaptation energy. The more stressors are experienced, the greater the drain on adaptation energy, the sooner the energy is used up. When no more adaptation energy is available, the third, 'exhaustion' stage is reached. Illness is likely. Then stimulated to excess the physiological adaptive process, designed to protect the body, may become maladaptive and produce pathological symptoms.

Stress and the immune system

Prolonged stimulation of the stress response produces higher than normal sustained levels of cortisol in the blood stream. Since one of the roles of cortisol in the stress response is to suppress the inflammatory reaction and the body's normal defence mechanisms, it will in the long-term have a dampening effect on the immune system. With its defences weakened, the body is much more likely to succumb to diseases, like infections, and to be unable to maintain a healthy level of functioning. This process explains why people are more susceptible to illness when experiencing much stress – for instance, the bride who develops a cold sore on her lip on her wedding day, or the supremely fit and healthy Olympic athlete who suddenly has a fever of 104 degrees with a severe upper respiratory tract infection on the eve of the final.

Table 9 Life changes with Life Change Units (LCUs)

Dr Richard Rahe's research shows that the more stressful the life changes experienced in a given period, the greater the incidence of illness; and the higher the score, the more serious the illness.

Life Event	Mean Value	Life Event	Mean Value
1 Death of spouse	100	24 Trouble with in-laws	29
2 Divorce	73	25 Outstanding personal achievement	28
3 Marital separation	65	26 Wife begins or stops work	26
4 Jail term	63	27 Begin or end school	26
5 Death of close family member	63	28 Change in living conditions	25
6 Personal injury or illness	53	29 Revision of personal habits	24
7 Marriage	50	30 Trouble with boss	23
8 Fired at work	47	31 Change in work hours or conditions	20
9 Marital reconciliation	45	32 Change in residence	20
10 Retirement	45	33 Change in school	20
11 Change in health of family member	44	34 Change in recreation	19
12 Pregnancy	40	35 Change in church activities	19
13 Sexual difficulties	39	36 Change in social activities	18
14 Gain of new family member	39	37 Lower mortgage or loan	17
15 Business readjustment	39	38 Change in sleeping habits	16
16 Change in financial state	38	39 Change in number of family get-togethers	15
17 Death of close friend	37	40 Change in eating habits	13
18 Change to different line of work	36	41 Vacation	13
19 Change in number of arguments with spouse	35	42 Minor violations of the law	11
20 High mortgage	31		
21 Foreclosure of mortgage or loan	30		
22 Change in responsibilities at work	29		
23 Son or daughter leaving home	29		

Source: Rahe in *Psychotropic Drug Response: Advances in Prediction*, May and Wittenborn, Illinois, (1969).

Stress and illness

Further light has been thrown recently by Dr Richard Rahe on the relationship between stressful life events and illness. Rahe drew up a table of forty-two 'life changes', each of which was allocated a value (a Life Change Unit – LCU) in terms of its stressfulness (see Table 9). Then, by following the medical and social history of a large number of people, he discovered a correlation between the amount of stress experienced from life changes (calculated as LCUs) and the amount of illness suffered during a specific period of between six months and two years. The more stressful life changes an individual experienced in a given period, the greater the incidence of illness; a cluster of significant life changes was followed by a cluster of diseases; the higher the stress score from life changes, the more serious the illness(es).

From Rahe's work, it seems clear that stress can cause changes in the body's functioning that may result in illness and disease. Since stress is not something that can be completely avoided, even if we wanted to, other ways of counteracting or balancing its effects must be found.

What to do about stress

To avoid squandering energy resources and to delay ageing, to cope with the stresses and strains of everyday life, to prevent illness and disease taking hold, this is what you should do:

* recognize stressful elements in your life

* adapt to, reduce or avoid stressful elements when possible

* be aware of your own personal stress reactions and individual arousal patterns

* acquire skills to manage the stress you experience in order to bring your state of arousal back to a comfortable and harmonious level

Knowing yourself

ARE YOU PRONE TO STRESS?

Stressful elements in your life can take any number of forms. Such an element may fall into the category of an environmental disaster, like a flood or hurricane, or a sudden unexpected event over which you have no control, like an accident or the death of someone close. For the most part, though, people, events, conditions and situations will be identified as stressful according to your ability to cope with them. Your coping ability will, in turn, be influenced by the beliefs and attitudes you hold, the assumptions you make and your perceptions. What you *think* is a vital factor in how you manage stress, and your physiological, biochemical and emotional response to stress will be affected by a combination of ideas, views, opinions, past experiences, expectations, values, needs, fears, judgements, evaluations and doctrines that make up your own unique way of thinking about the world.

A number of personality characteristics or behaviour patterns are associated with an individual's ability to cope with stress.

TYPE A BEHAVIOUR

Typically, Type A behaviour is manifested by the workaholic who works long hours constantly to a deadline, takes work home, does not take proper holidays, cannot relax, is irritable and often shows hostility, is self-disciplined and has high, often unrealistic standards. Individuals manifesting Type A behaviour seem to create stress and, one could say, thrive upon it.

Conversely, Type Bs are the sane people of the world. Placid, calm and flexible, they plan and organize their lives without angst or hassle. They enjoy life for its own sake and can truly relax without needing or wanting to compete. Interestingly, only about 1 in 10 individuals are true Type Bs – a creative Type B might be a craftsman or woman or possibly an artist. In the middle are the Type ABs who show a healthy, balanced attitude to life, are able to establish good relationships and cope effectively with stress, but who can 'rev up' and 'go for it' when they want to.

It may be that Type As 'need' the effects of large amounts of circulating stress hormones to function at a very high level of arousal, for which the reward is that a great deal gets done. But the price exacted for this overworking of the system is an increased risk of coronary heart disease. Type A individuals are more than twice as likely to suffer from heart attacks as people who do not manifest this behaviour pattern. According to Dr Meyer Friedman who, with Dr Ray Rosenman, did some of the original work in this area, 'the toxic element . . . is the *struggle*'.

Fortunately, with conscientious re-apprai-

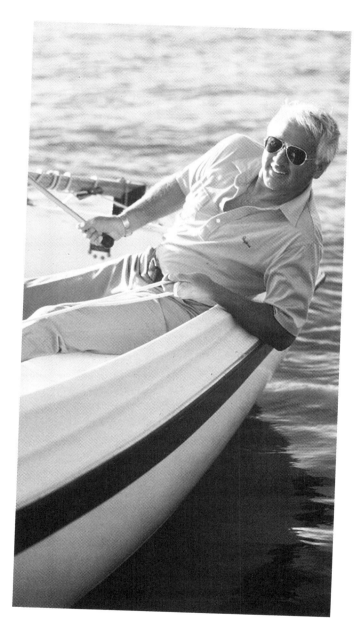

Taking up a sporting activity can provide an 'escape route' for relieving stress

Table 10 Find out what behaviour type you are

Each of us lies somewhere along the line between the two extremes. For example, most of us are neither the most competitive nor the least competitive person we know. Fill in the circle where you think you belong between these two extremes.

1.	Never late _____ ○○○○○○○○○○	Casual about appointments ____	
2.	Very competitive _____ ○○○○○○○○○○	Not competitive _____	
3.	Anticipate what others are going to say (nod, interrupt, finish for them) ○○○○○○○○○○	Good listener, hear others out ___	
4.	Always rushed _____ ○○○○○○○○○○	Never feel rushed, even under pressure __ __	
5.	Impatient when waiting _____ ○○○○○○○○○○	Can wait patiently _____	
6.	Go 'all out' _____ ○○○○○○○○○○	Casual _____	
7.	Try to do too many things at once, think about what you are going to do next ○○○○○○○○○○	Take things one at a time _____	
8.	Emphatic in speech (may pound desk) ○○○○○○○○○○	Slow, deliberate talker _____	
9.	Want good job to be recognised by others ○○○○○○○○○○	Only care about satisfying yourself no matter what others may think	
10.	Fast (eating, talking, etc.) _____ ○○○○○○○○○○	Slow doing things _____	
11.	Hard driving _____ ○○○○○○○○○○	Easy going _____	
12.	Sit on feelings _____ ○○○○○○○○○○	Express feelings _____	
13.	Few interests outside work _____ ○○○○○○○○○○	Many interests _____	
14.	Ambitious _____ ○○○○○○○○○○	Satisfied with job _____	
		Total	

Count the circles from the right up to your 'filled in' circle and add up your total score.

Results

Score		
14–30	Ultra B – extremely rare. If he or she exists at all, the individual is probably too relaxed to do the questionnaire!	
31–60	Type B – very sane; personality and lifestyle definitely not a danger to health.	
61–70	Type AB – nice, healthy balance. Health probably not at risk.	
71–80	Type A – showing elements of damaging Type A behaviour. Personality and lifestyle may begin to put health at risk.	
81–100	High Type A – personality and lifestyle definitely in danger of putting health at risk.	
101–120	Extreme Type A – real go-getters, highly competitive. Almost certain to put their health at risk.	
120+	Extremely rare; no such individual has been discovered in current research.	

Studies carried out by Steve Regis, a stress management consultant, on large work groups has shown that senior management groups fall into the Type A category as a norm, scoring an average of nearly 80. Other groups, for instance local government workers and those in business, had a lower average score of 75 with a spread between 60 and 85. These scores in these latter groups are typical of most people, with women generally scoring slightly lower than men. Within each group there are individuals who scored much higher and much lower than the average for that group. For instance, one director of a company scored 112 – a very high score that indicates that he may be at risk of a premature heart attack. Another more phlegmatic senior executive, however, scored only 60.

If you have the kind of drive that puts you amongst the high Type As, it would be impossible to change your personality completely. In any case, it is likely that your success in a highly competitive world is due, in part, to the forceful elements in your character and it would be undesirable to alter them radically. You can, though, train yourself to switch them off when they are unnecessary, inappropriate or simply a habit that may put you at risk and distress your family and colleagues. For instance, in particular when driving, gardening, doing chores, socializing or on holiday, it is important to eliminate the competitive element and to learn to enjoy activities like these for their own sake.

sal and a burgeoning self-awareness of old be-haviour patterns, harmful habits can be changed and the risk of heart attacks significantly reduced. As one reformed Type A said, 'Now I realize that if I'm late for that meeting, the world isn't going to come to a stop.'

There is a spectrum of possible behaviour types from ultra-Bs to extreme-As. Table 10 will give you some idea of where on the scale you lie.

LOCUS OF CONTROL

Some people have a tendency to feel at the mercy of 'the slings and arrows of outrageous fortune' and may feel trapped in a stressful way of life they perceive to be largely outside their own jurisdiction. For them, taking possession of their own fate can be very problematical.

An important issue for such individuals is where they experience the *locus of control*. Someone with an internal locus of control feels in control of his/her life, responsible for the decisions and actions taken, and able to change circumstances should they become too stressful; an individual whose locus of control is external tends to feel that he or she has little influence on circumstances and is unable to influence what luck or fate has in store. The externally orientated person is prone to feeling victimized and his/her passivity stands in the way of making adjustments to alter or avoid stressful situations.

Fortunately, most of us experience life somewhere in the middle of the internal/external locus of control scale but it will vary according to the degree to which we are cop-ing with the stress in our lives and what the stressors are. Recognizing your own propensity and coping capacity at any particular time allows you to make appropriate choices with respect to jobs, careers and relationships.

HARDINESS AND MASTERY

Hardiness is thought to make a person particularly resilient to stressful life events. Three traits typical of the 'hardy' personality have been described by Dr Kobasa, an American psychologist: *commitment*, meaning complete involvement with whatever task is undertaken; *challenge*, meaning flexibility, an acceptance of change, and a willingness to shift and revise; *control* which, like the internal locus of control, indicates a sense of being in charge of the outcome of events. Hardy types tend to experience stressful events as potential opportunities for change even when they may seem unpleasant, knowing that they have all the resources they need to cope. Such individuals have a sense of mastery over their fate which empowers them so that they experience life as a 'flow' not as a battle. They swim down the river with the tide, not up it against the stream. Naturally, life seems less stressful as a result.

Dr Kobasa also found that physical exercise provided an additional factor in these individuals' stress-resistant patterns. She discovered that both hardiness and exercise acted as buffers in the relationship between stress and illness, and that the buffering effects of hardiness and exercise are additive: persons who were high on the hardiness scale *and* who exercised were the healthiest.

Coping skills

A critical first step in the management of stress is to observe the way in which an event or person is perceived and then to make a re-appraisal based on logic and reasoning rather than the habitual, deeply rooted, automatic emotional reactions of the past. This approach is known as *cognitive restructuring* and is utilized in a number of psychotherapeutic approaches, including reality therapy (William Glasser), cognitive behaviour therapy (Aaron Beck), rational emotive therapy (Albert Ellis) and transactional analysis (Eric Berne).

The re-appraisal involves identifying distortions in the way an event is perceived and in consciously changing that perception. For instance, a request to go to the boss's office for an unscheduled meeting may produce a typical panic reaction and speculation: 'What have I done wrong? . . . he's going to fire me . . . or at least tear me off a strip for something . . .' These negative thoughts predominate and result in a full-blown fight or flight response with a dry mouth, thumping heart beat, sweaty palms and churning stomach. Using the skill of cognitive restructuring, this person would reassess and *reframe* the situation with constructive self-talk based on what is real, not what is imagined or feared.

STRESS WARNING SIGNALS

Professor Cary Cooper, who has worked extensively in the field of stress, suggests that if you are going through a period of considerable discomfort due to stress, there may be not just one source of stress in your life but a number of linked incidents forming a 'stress-chain'.

In order to understand these linked incidents, Professor Cooper proposes that you keep a record or diary of your personal stress warning signals – such as headaches, stomach pains, muscle tension, depression, anxiety or a strong desire to escape a situation – which can then be used to create an action plan to minimize or eliminate the stress factors.

Your stress diary would include:

* day of week, and time

* the incident (what happened)

* people involved

* what you did

* your physical and/or emotional feelings

* what you should have done

The diary should be kept at the end of each day for several weeks, at the end of which you can evaluate which people and events seemed to be most stressful. Was there a pattern discernible? Did you experience most stress at home or at work? Were you subjected to time pressures, uncertainties, overload, lack of support? Were relationships with your spouse, children, in-laws, boss, partner implicated?

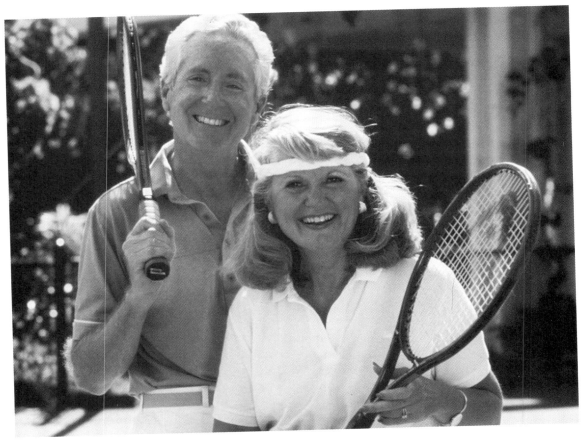

Regular exercise is thought to have an anti-depressant effect

ALTERNATIVE STRATEGIES

Having identified the sources of stress, it is possible to think of alternative strategies to help you cope and to minimize future stress. Some strategies may involve actual changes in practical arrangements at work or at home, others may involve changing your own behaviour and acquiring personal skills like learning to relax or to be more self-assertive.

Low-stress lifestyle

Most of us are familiar with the stress-relieving effects of alcohol before an important event like a wedding; a small dram of whisky has been known to calm the nerves and sharpen the wits before an important interview. But the regular use of palliatives like tobacco, coffee and alcohol as a way of coping

with a highly stressed life can be harmful. Becoming aware of those aspects of your lifestyle that generate high stress enables you to do something about them or your reaction to them before negative consequences occur.

Karl Albrecht, who wrote *Stress and the Manager*, identified a number of elements of a low-stress lifestyle, many of which are based on straightforward common sense. For instance, someone who experiences difficult relationships with family, lover, boss, etc., could relieve the stress by having 'escape routes' (other than the pub), allowing occasional separation and relaxation, like the potting shed, a sport or an interest. He or she would also make sure, when entering new friendships, that they were low on stress, not likely to prove difficult and perhaps harmful.

A low-stress lifestyle, according to Albrecht, would include eating well, using alcohol in moderation, keeping physically fit and engaging in a variety of activities that bring satisfaction and pleasure, including enjoying a 'full and exuberant sex life', the latter being more typically stress relieving than low stress.

The essence of a relatively stress-free existence, or at least one in which the stress is manageable and not overwhelming, seems to be to achieve a well-balanced, positive outlook. It includes saying 'No' to extra work or commitments when you already have enough on your plate, being flexible, seeing options and alternatives when difficult decisions present themselves, and rewarding yourself when a demanding or complex project has been brought to a satisfactory conclusion.

STRESS AND EXERCISE

Aerobically fit men and women, according to studies carried out in the USA by Drs Crews and Landers, are able to cope more effectively with stress than unfit people. Aerobically fit individuals recover more rapidly, physiologically as well as psychologically, from emotional stress; they have a reduced stress response regardless of the type of psychological or social stressor; they are less likely to become physically ill or depressed than unfit individuals under similar amounts of stress, because the fit person may be in a better immunological condition to fight off disease, and they perceive their lives as less stressful. They sleep more restfully and experience improved self-esteem.

Regular exercise can bring beneficial mood changes and effects on the personality. The short-term benefits experienced for a few hours after a work-out are related to enhanced mood – a general sense of well-being, of feeling good, often described as an 'afterglow'. Long-term participation can result in decreased symptoms of anxiety and depression.

The psychological effects of exercise are not fully understood but may be related to the increased secretion of neurotransmitters in the brain, the endorphins, which are 'morphine-like' compounds that reduce the sensation of pain and produce euphoria. Another hypothesis implicates the effect of a raised body temperature that occurs during vigorous exercise, which, like the alleged health benefits of taking sauna baths, is thought to produce a sensation of well-being. This may help to explain the 'high' you may feel when you have a fever, and the anxiety-relieving effect of a hot bath. Furthermore, it has been proposed that a 'pyrogenic' factor, if one exists, may alter the activity of the brain neurotransmitters, noradrenalin and serotonin, which are known to be disturbed in depression. Regular exercise is associated with raised levels of these two brain chemicals and, therefore, could have an anti-depressant effect.

Quite apart from the obvious physical and psychological benefits, exercise can relieve stress by distracting you from the stressful conditions in your life, and by providing a channel for pent-up anger and frustration. It can also provide a vehicle for social support, interaction and companionship. Sometimes, as adults, we forget how to play and we forego our right to have fun.

It could be argued that exercise itself is a form of stress, especially vigorous games and highly competitive sports that, in an already overstressed individual, may become just one more stressor. But the experts do not all agree. Many people enjoy competition for its own sake and would find exercising intolerable without it. An individual who has an overwhelming compulsion to win at all costs clearly has a problem which has little to do with the physical activity. But, for some people, the element of competition adds a *raison d'être* that makes exercise a pleasure not a chore. In order to become a habit, an exercise programme has to be enjoyable.

STRESS AND RELAXATION

When a person is stressed, the sympathetic nervous system is stimulated. The effect on the individual is a feeling of 'arousal'. A certain optimum level of arousal is essential when you aim to achieve a specific result or produce a desirable performance. It is said that you have to feel some nervousness in order to give of your best, whether it is in an examination, a competition, a stage performance or any other goal-orientated activity.

If you are under-aroused, you are likely to perform below your best. Equally, if you are over-aroused and feeling 'up-tight', your performance may be impaired. An hypothesis relating performance and arousal has been expressed graphically by Yerkes and Dobson and referred to as the 'inverted U hypothesis' (see Figure 6). This shows performance and arousal both increasing in a more or less linear fashion up to a certain optimum point after which further arousal causes performance to get worse and the line of the graph slopes downwards. An individual who is feeling 'under stress' and performing poorly but who responds by working even longer hours, trying even harder to make up for lost ground and who becomes anxious and exhausted, is showing signs of over-arousal.

The body needs to be able to 'switch off', to relax, recover and recuperate. To produce this state, the 'burner' of the sympathetic nervous system must be turned down whilst the parasympathetic nervous system is stimulated. The effect on the body is practically the opposite to that of sympathetic stimulation; namely, heart rate and respiration are slower, blood pressure is lower, muscle tension decreases, stress hormone levels decrease and blood flow to the extremities increases.

Cats switch from the stressed fight or flight state to one of relaxation and recovery naturally when they stretch out in a warm place after a spot of stalking and hunting. Human beings also have the capacity to illicit this 'relaxation response' but, for many of us, this natural ability has been lost or forgotten. It can, however, be re-learnt using any one of a number of techniques such as progressive muscle relaxation, autogenic training, meditation, yoga, self-hypnosis, biofeedback, visualization and mental imagery. For the best results, these techniques are best learnt with the help of specialized teachers who can guide and advise during the training period. An experienced teacher will advise on the best techniques to adopt. Once learnt, they can be used regularly to induce a general feeling of relaxation and well-being.

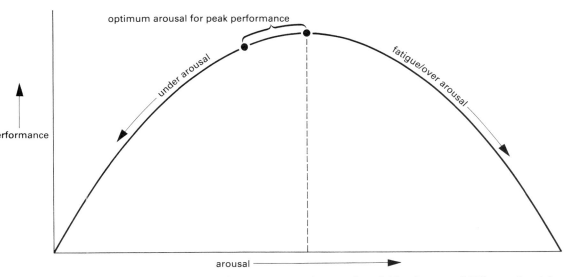

Figure 6 *How performance and stress arousal are related (the inverted U hypothesis)*

It is possible to begin to learn to relax using Progressive Muscle Relaxation (of Professor Edmund Jacobson) that uses the contrasting sensation of contraction and relaxation of muscles to relieve muscle tension.

It is important to remember to breathe properly whilst doing the exercise. Ideally, you should breathe normally without co-ordinating your in and out breaths with the tensing and relaxing of the muscles. If this is difficult to begin with, breathe in when you tense the muscle and then breathe out with a long, slow breath when you let go of the tension and relax. Don't contract muscles too hard or for too long – just hard enough and long enough (no more than 5 or 6 seconds) to feel the tension in the muscles before relaxing them and feeling the contrast.

Progressive muscle relaxation is not suitable for everyone; in particular, it is not recommended for people with high blood pressure, as tensing the muscles raises the blood pressure momentarily. Also, some individuals may paradoxically experience an *increase* in tension using this method. For these people,

and for those who wish to progress to a state of deeper relaxation after using progressive muscle relaxation, the focusing technique is recommended. For this, take up a similar position lying down on your back and prepare in the same way as described below for progressive muscle relaxation.

1. Lie flat on your back in a warm, quiet, comfortable place. Release any tight clothing such as a belt or tie, and remove spectacles. Rest your arms, slightly bent at the elbows, by the side of your body (not touching it) with the palms down, fingers relaxed and loose. Legs are slightly apart; a pillow can be placed under the knees to support them if desired. The head can also be supported by a thin pillow.

2. Close your eyes. Take some deep, slow breaths and as you breathe out through the mouth, let out a sigh and be aware of *letting go.*

3. Then follow the programme.

PROGRESSIVE MUSCLE RELAXATION

First of all, squeeze both hands into fists, as hard as you can. Keep squeezing and notice the pattern of tension. Hold for 5 or 6 seconds. Now let both hands go limp and relaxed. Notice the difference between the tense feeling and the relaxation you feel now. Now clench your fists again, bring your fists up to your shoulders and contract your upper arms to notice the pattern of tension, hold for 5 or 6 seconds and – relax. Let both your arms become completely relaxed.

Shoulders

Raise both shoulders up to your ears. Hold this position and notice the way it clenches your muscles. Feel the tension produced. And now – relax.

Now pull your shoulders forwards and contract the muscles of the upper chest. Hold and now – relax.

Now pull your shoulders back and feel the tension in the upper back. Hold your shoulders back. And now – relax.

Let the whole of your arms and upper body relax. Let the whole of your upper body become more and more relaxed.

Face

Now let's concentrate on the face. Begin by raising your eyebrows as high as they can. Feel the tension in your forehead and relax.

Now try and bring your eyebrows together over the bridge of your nose, causing vertical lines of tension above the nose.

Some of you may be recognizing habitual patterns of tension which you feel every day.

And now relax. Let your forehead completely relax.

Screw up your eyes, as tight as you can. Hold for a few seconds. Now relax your eyes.

Now for the cheek muscles. First of all, contract the left cheek, pulling your mouth sideways in a lopsided grin. Feel the tension on this side of your face. Now relax.

Contract the right cheek. Hold the tension. And now relax. Let both cheeks become more and more relaxed. Feel your mouth relax.

Clench your teeth to contract the muscles of the jaw. Become aware of this pattern of tension. Again, many of you may recognize a familiar source of discomfort.

Now relax again – allow the whole face to become relaxed and smooth, allowing the tension to flow away and the muscles to relax more and more.

Focus again on your shoulders and arms and become aware of the feelings of relaxation here too.

Concentrate on the feelings of relaxation in the whole of your face, shoulders and upper body.

Every time you breathe out, let your body become more and more relaxed. All tensions should now be drained away.

Now bring your mind back to the room and away from the body. Flutter your eyelids and then slowly open your eyes. Have a good stretch and wake up.

FOCUSING TECHNIQUE

Here we are going to be concentrating on different areas of the body, working upwards from the toes to the head and becoming aware of each area in turn.

Begin by becoming aware of your

right big toe	right fourth toe
right second toe	and right little
right third toe	toe

Become aware of the

sole of your right foot	right calf and
the top of your right	right knee
foot	the whole of
your right heel	your lower
right ankle	right leg

Become aware of your

upper right thigh	the whole of
lower right thigh	your right leg
right buttock	from top to
right hip and	bottom

Now repeat the same awareness techniques for your left foot and leg.

Now become aware of your

right thumb	right fourth
right index finger	finger and
right middle finger	right little finger

Become aware of your

right upper hand	right elbow and
the palm of your	the whole of
right hand	your right
your right wrist	lower arm
right forearm	

Become aware of your

right upper arm	from shoulder
right shoulder and	to fingertips
the whole right arm	

Now repeat the same awareness techniques for your left hand and arm.

Become aware of the

back of your neck	the top of your
the back of your	head
head	

Become aware of your

left forehead	right cheek
right forehead	nose
left eyebrow	upper lip
right eyebrow	lower lip
left eye	chin
right eye	throat and your
left cheek	whole face

Become aware of your

right upper chest	abdomen
left upper chest	upper back
lower chest	lower back
waist	whole torso

Become aware of your

whole right leg	head and face
whole left leg	torso
whole right arm	whole body
whole left arm	

Every time you breathe out, let your body become more and more relaxed. Let all tension drain away. Allow yourself to become more and more relaxed.

Become aware of your whole body.

Slowly come back to the present, to the room you are in. Flutter your eyelids and allow yourself to open your eyes. Become fully awake once more.

ADDITIONAL REMARKS

It is important to keep your mind on the part of the body on which you are focusing. If your thoughts wander – and this is quite common – gently bring them back. As far as possible, be the passive observer, noticing everything that happens but without making judgements or evaluations. With this passively aware attitude, you can bring your wandering thoughts back to concentrate on your body without becoming irritated or impatient with yourself. Ideally, these relaxation techniques should be practised each day, better still twice a day for maximum benefit, either before eating or an hour or so after a meal.

Read the instructions through carefully several times before starting. Alternatively, record the instructions on an audio-cassette in a slow, fairly monotonous voice and practise the technique listening to the tape.

For individuals who want to explore relaxation and its effects on stress and health in more depth, a course of Autogenic Training with a qualified teacher is strongly recommended.

AUTOGENIC TRAINING (AT) – WHAT IS IT?

'Autogenic' means generated from the self. AT is a system which brings profound relaxation and stress release. It consists of six simple mental exercises learnt over a period of about eight weeks, which allow the mind to be calm and the body completely relaxed, by 'turning down' the sympathetic nervous system's stress reponse and allowing the relaxing, re-cuperative, regenerative effects of the para-sympathetic nervous system to take over (see page 90). The result is that the usual state of over-arousal and stress in the body and mind that most of us experience most of the time, is replaced with one of relaxation, peacefulness and calm.

In addition to the calming effect on the mental state, known as the autogenic state (an altered state of consciousness akin to certain meditational states), AT has a profound regulatory and rebalancing effect on the body's physiological functions that, with practice, results in a lower heart rate, lower blood pressure and a boost to the immune system. As a result, a wide range of disorders can be affected beneficially, including hypertension, asthma, irritable bowel, colitis, peptic and duodenal ulcers, arthritis, muscular pain and tension, migraine headaches, allergic skin reactions and constipation. A reliance on drugs to treat these conditions can diminish significantly with AT practice.

In addition, psychological problems such as anxiety states, insomnia, unresolved grief reactions, bulimia, the mental state accompanying ME and disturbances due to stress, can be helped by AT, either directly or to support and enhance progress with other therapies.

Equally, it is not necessary to have symptoms to benefit from AT. Individuals wishing to improve their performance, like Olympic athletes, dancers or musicians, or to improve work efficiency like business people and other professionals, or to mobilize creativity like artists or teachers, have all benefited from practising AT. American and Russian astronauts learnt AT before journeying into space.

STRESS AND TOUCHING

The British, it appears, touch one another less than people of most other nations. Observation of couples talking in coffee shops in several different countries showed that the rate of touching varied from 180 touches per hour in Puerto Rico to none at all in London. An attempt was made to quantify the value of touching at a medical conference in Canada; it was proposed that four hugs a day acts as an antidote for depression, eight contributes greatly to mental stability and twelve cuddles a day could promote real psychological well-being (assuming that the hugs were welcome and from someone 'near and dear').

The skin is the largest sensory organ of the body. Just as melodious music and beautiful landscapes can act as antidotes to stress through sensory stimulation of our ears and eyes, touching, stroking and massaging the skin can have a significant stress-relieving effect.

STRESS AND HUMOUR

Norman Cousins, author of *Anatomy of an Illness*, was suffering from a crippling disease that affected all his joints and muscles. He was completely bedridden, unable to move even his fingers. He was told by his doctor that his chances of recovery were extremely remote, less than one in 500. The prognosis was very bad indeed. Not prepared to accept this miserable life sentence, Cousins literally laughed himself well by watching comedy films, like the Marx Brothers and programmes like 'Candid Camera' and reading humorous books.

Within a matter of days, his condition started to improve; eventually he was able to return to work. Is this a joke? Not at all. After each bout of laughing, Cousins's blood tests showed a slight improvement until, eventually, his disease remitted and he recovered.

According to Dr Paul Ekman, an American psychologist, there is more to smiling than meets the eye. The act of flexing facial muscles into expressions of joy may produce effects in the brain and autonomic nervous system characteristic of this emotion. Blood flow and brain temperature are altered so that chemicals in the brain (neurotransmitters) are affected. In other words, acting out or mimicking an emotion without actually feeling it can have a physical effect.

SUMMARY

If stress was re-labelled as stimuli, we could avoid the negative connotations that the word 'stress' evokes. Stimuli are to be welcomed; they represent the cut and thrust of life, the 'ups and downs' without which life would have a boring, if safe, sameness and predictability. The key to health and well-being, as mentioned in Chapter 3, is being able to meet the broadest spectrum of possible challenges – physical, mental and emotional. In other words, to be able to cope with and manage the wide variety of stimuli or stresses that life throws up.

EIGHT

Exercise

It was not so long ago that human beings were nomads and hunters; our ancestors needed to have considerable strength, speed and agility in order to survive. It is only in relatively recent times, with the enormous strides that have been made technologically, resulting in motorized transport and a plethora of labour-saving devices, that a drastic reduction has occurred in the amount of physical activity performed in daily life both at work and in the home. Most people today living in industrialized countries are unfit. The drop in fitness levels has been accompanied by a simultaneous rise in death and disability due to cardiovascular disease in these populations. One can say without much fear of contradiction that our present sedentary lifestyle has considerable drawbacks so far as the health of the nation is concerned.

I am sure our grandmothers and grandfathers, manacled to the scrubbing brush, washboard, mangle and carpet beater, would envy our washing machines, dishwashers and vacuum cleaners, and the leisure these machines have brought us. But for the most part, we have taken our increased leisure time lying down. We have failed to replace the enforced physical labour that typified work until a couple of generations ago, with voluntary physical activity in out-of-work hours. It is understandable that our generation and that of our parents assumed a more sedentary lifestyle as improved standards of living meant that working conditions both in the house and at work became much less physically demanding. Physical activity in the home and at work was associated with hard, tiring, often backbreaking work and, for most people, the less

of that the better. And who was to know that the price some would have to pay for our modern-day luxurious inertia would be prematurely stiff joints, weakness, disability and disease?

Fortunately, all is not lost. The benefits of a physically active life can be yours for the taking – no previous experience necessary. The first step in realizing the benefits of adopting a more active lifestyle, namely, the easing of effort in everyday activities and the lessening of fatigue, is to build up an awareness of using the body to extend its physical capabilities in everyday activities. For instance, simply moving around more can have a surprisingly positive influence on our state of physical fitness, e.g. stretching for something on a top shelf, bending to pick something up, playing with the children, enjoying walking more, stretching, walking up and down stairs instead of taking the lift or escalator. If you have been a 'couch potato' for some time, any amount of increase in physical activity will contribute towards an improvement in your fitness level, however small. Those jobs that have seemed so hard and required such a great effort, tasks that perhaps you had to stop halfway through because of the early onset of extreme fatigue, will be completed with unaccustomed ease and in less time.

Engaging in more vigorous aerobic exercise such as brisk walking, running, cycling or swimming, involving the rhythmic use of the larger muscle groups, can substantially delay the onset of a multiplicity of ageing effects described in Chapter 3. At a recent conference of world experts, the following conclusion was reached: 'Exercise training in the fifth and

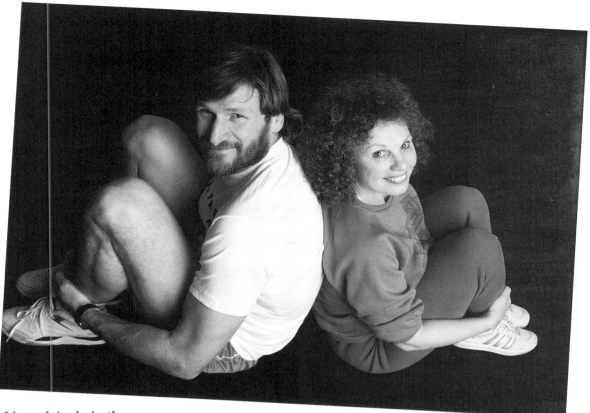

Liz and Andy in the gym

sixth decades of life [i.e. forties-plus] may allev-iate this decline [in capacity], but more im-portantly will induce a functional gain, equivalent to as much as 10–15 years in many individuals.' In other words, in your mid-forties you could regain the physical power, speed and strength you had when thirty-five or so, if you take part in regular exercise.

To achieve these results effectively, a train-ing programme to improve stamina, to streng-then muscles and improve or maintain flexib-ility of joint movements is required. After only a few weeks of a regular exercise programme, there is a 'training effect' and you will ex-perience a general improvement in physical capacity. Your step will lighten as you bound up the stairs and you will be able to have a con-versation without puffing as soon as you arrive. No more 'Just let me get my breath back.' For training to occur, the effort you put into the exercise needs to be a little greater than that to which you are normally accustomed. Even if you have been com-pletely sedentary up until now, you will show an improvement in physical capacity with even the lowest intensity of exercise. For some, simply getting up to change TV chan-nels will be enough to start the process. Equally, if you have been quite active, but you want to be fitter, you will need to engage in an exercise programme that is sufficiently demanding to extend you physically.

The improvement in physical fitness will depend on the intensity, duration and fre-quency of the activity. As the effects of train-ing accumulate over a period of weeks or months, you will have to work harder, and/or longer and perhaps more often in order to sus-tain the training effects. If you stop exercising the gains will gradually be lost and your body will eventually return to its pre-training state. But then, you could always start again.

How to exercise

What kind of exercise? How often should I do it? How hard and for how long? The answers to these questions depend on a number of criteria. Ideally, an exercise programme should be tailored to the individual to take into account his or her physical condition, age, state of health, lifestyle, goals, motivation and access to facilities. What are your reasons for exercising? Are you exercising for health reasons, physical fitness, body shape, weight control, self-image, to feel good, to enhance your mood, companionship, competitiveness, skill mastery or because it's Tuesday? Whatever your personal agenda may be, a fitness programme needs to *fit* into your life, otherwise it is unlikely to survive.*

If you are starting to plan an exercise training programme for the first time, it is a good idea to remember that, in general, slower is better than faster, low intensity better than high, and, above all, 'more' is not always 'better'. Even the word 'programme' can be off-putting, conjuring up images of vigorous training sessions in the gym and serious preparation for major events like marathons or the like. In fact, an exercise programme can simply mean a regular, daily, two-mile walk with the dog. It is important that the initial exercise experience is enjoyable, refreshing, and not too demanding either physically, or in terms of time.

Exercise programmes have a notoriously high drop-out rate. Nearly 50% of vigorous exercisers quit within a year, whereas the drop-out rate from *moderate* activity is half that. With a gradual, softly-softly approach, you are much more likely to have a positive attitude towards the programme, and to develop an enthusiastic commitment to staying with it.

What kind of exercise?

A well-rounded exercise programme for total fitness should include the following:

1. ***Aerobic activities***, including fast walking, jogging/running, swimming, cycling, vigorous games, dancing, stair-climbing, to develop and maintain cardio-respiratory fitness and weight control.

2. ***Strength and muscular endurance activities***, such as weight-training, strengthening exercises (like press-ups and sit-ups) and circuit-training, to strengthen muscles, maintain muscle tone and bone density, and protect against injury and low-back pain.

3. ***Flexibility exercises***, such as stretching and joint mobilization, to develop and maintain an optimal range of joint movement to prevent poor posture, fatigue and injury, and to promote agility.

All three kinds of exercise are equally important to all-round fitness.

*It is strongly recommended that anyone intending to increase substantially their level of physical activity through a fitness programme should consult his or her doctor before doing so.

WARM-UP/WARM-DOWN

At the start of an exercise session, it is essential to warm-up in order to avoid injury and to prepare your muscles for vigorous exercise. A warm-up exercise is any exercise that is sufficiently energetic to raise the heart rate 15 to 20 beats per minute and to increase the blood flow to the large muscle groups of the legs and arms. The muscles literally warm-up. Brisk walking, slow jogging are good for this purpose. Alternatively, the two exercises shown below are also very good.

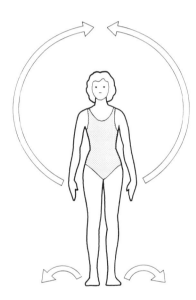

Jumping Jacks

Stand upright with your feet together and your arms hanging loosely by your sides. Jump into an astride position, raising your arms straight out to the side above your head. In a continuous movement, jump back to the original position with feet together and arms lowered straight down the side to vertical. Repeat this continuously for 1–2 minutes.

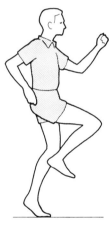

Running on the spot

Run in one place on the balls of your feet for 1–2 minutes.

STRETCHING EXERCISES

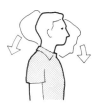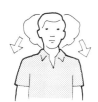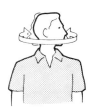

Neck stretch

Having warmed up your muscles and raised your heart rate moderately with the previous exercises, it is advisable to stretch those muscles and joints that you will be using in the aerobic activity to follow. For instance, if you are going to run, you need to stretch the muscles of your thighs, calves and ankles. If you are going to swim you need to pay attention to your arms, shoulders, neck and trunk as well.

In the warm-down period at the end of the session, you can use stretching exercises to increase joint mobility and range of movement whilst the tissues are still warm and can be stretched without fear of tearing.

Once or twice a week it is advisable to spend a longer period of time, say 20 minutes plus, on stretching and to go through the complete programme of stretching exercises illustrated here. As a result, you will increase your agility considerably, avoid stiffening of the joints and stay limber longer.

Stand with feet apart and arms hanging loosely by sides. Bend head back, look at ceiling. Hold for 3 seconds. Bend head forwards, chin on chest, hold for 3 seconds. Return head to normal position. Tip head over to right – hold for 3 seconds. Return to normal. Tip head over to left – hold for 3 seconds. Return to normal. Turn head to right as if to look over right shoulder – hold for 3 seconds. Return to normal. Turn head to left – hold for 3 seconds. Return to normal position.

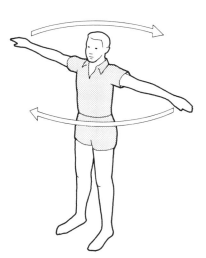

For back, sides and shoulders

Stand with feet apart and pointed forward. Raise arms to shoulder level. Keeping feet flat on the floor, twist to right. Do this 3 times to the right and 3 to the left. Repeat 10 times.

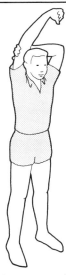

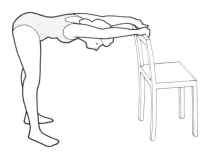

Grasp the back of a chair (made secure).
Slightly bend your knees and slowly lean
forward letting head and chest hang down.
Feel the tension in the muscles for 30 seconds
(building to 60 seconds). Repeat twice.

For shoulders
and sides

*Stand upright, feet apart, right arm raised
above your head, left hand grasping right
upper arm just above your right elbow behind
your head. With left hand, pull right arm
towards left side behind your head. Feel the
stretch in your right shoulder. Hold for 10
seconds. Repeat on the other side.*

For bottom and backs
of the legs

*With feet apart and
hands on hips, slowly
bend forward – from
the hips not the waist
– keeping the back
flat. Slowly return to
the upright position.
Repeat 10 times.*

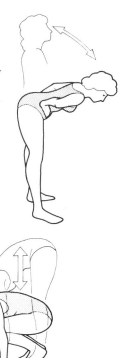

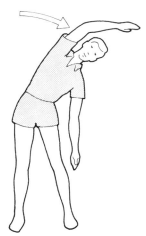

*Stand upright, feet more than shoulder width
apart, right arm raised above your head, the
other at your side. Keeping both feet flat,
bend to the left, right arm stretching
overhead. Repeat to the left. Repeat 5 times,
building up to 10.*

*With feet together, crouch down with knees
bent and hands flat on floor. Straighten knees
as far as possible with hands still flat on floor.
Knees do not have to be completely straight.
Do not bounce. Hold position for 10 seconds.
Repeat 3 times.*

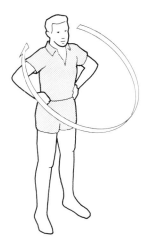

For abdomen

With feet apart and hands on hips, bend to the left. Rotate to the forward position, then to the right and return to the upright. Do this twice to the left and twice to the right. Repeat 10 times.

This exercise also stretches the abdominal muscles.

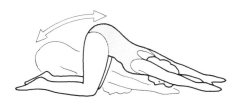

For lower back

Kneel, sitting back on your feet. Lean forward, arms stretched in front of you, palms face down on the floor. Slowly rock back until buttocks touch heels, rounding your back. Repeat 10 times.

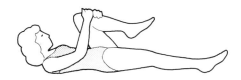

Lie on your back with legs extended. Lift and bend one leg, grasping the knee. Keep other leg flat. Pull the knee up to your chest. Repeat with the other leg. Repeat 10 times.

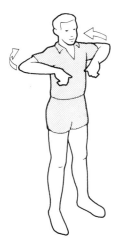

For shoulders and chest

Either stand with feet slightly apart or kneel. Raise arms to shoulder level. With elbows bent, push arms backwards and return. Repeat 10 times, building up to 15.

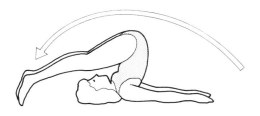

For lower back and hamstrings

This is more strenuous than the previous two exercises. Lie on your back with your legs bent. Keeping your knees together, slowly bring them over your head. Straighten legs and touch the floor with your toes. Hold for two counts and return to starting position. Repeat 5 times, building up to 10.

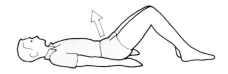

For hips, bottom and abdomen (the bottom-firmer)

Lie on back, feet a little apart, knees bent, arms flat on floor by your sides. Lift pelvis off floor so that the front of your body is in a straight line from shoulders to knees. Clench the buttocks together and hold for 10 seconds. Repeat 5 times.

For thighs and legs

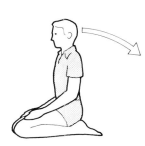

Kneel on the floor with legs touching. Sit back on your heels, arms resting on the front of your thighs. Let your trunk rock backwards until you feel a stretch in the muscles in the front of your thighs. Hold it for 5 seconds. Repeat 5 times.

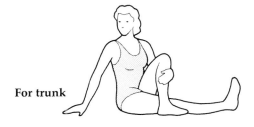

For trunk

Sit on the floor with your right leg stretched out in front and your left knee bent with your left foot on the right side of your right knee. Your left hand holds your left leg just below the knee and your right hand is flat on the floor by your right side. Keeping your trunk upright, twist to the right, looking over your right shoulder and reaching backwards on the floor with your right hand. Hold for 10 seconds. Repeat on the other side.

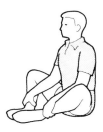

For groin

Sit with soles of feet pressed together, knees bent outward. Grasp the inside of your calves and pull upper body as near as possible to your feet. Hold for 30 seconds (building up to 60 seconds). Repeat once for a few sessions, then twice.

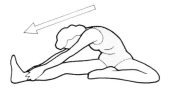

For hamstrings (backs of legs and thighs)

Sit on the floor with one leg straight out in front of you. The sole of the other foot should be touching the inner thigh. Bend forward and try to touch the knee of the extended leg with your forehead. Hold for 30 seconds (building up to 60 seconds). Repeat with the other leg. Repeat once for a few sessions, then twice.

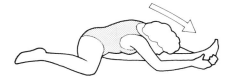

Sit on the floor, one leg straight out in front of you. Bend the other leg backwards, so you are in a hurdling position. Bend forward and try to touch your knee with your forehead. Hold for 30 seconds (building up to 60 seconds). Repeat once for a few sessions, then twice.

This exercise is more strenuous than the previous one and shouldn't be attempted by anyone with knee problems.

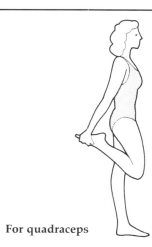

For quadraceps

Stand upright with feet slightly apart, arms by your sides. Bend your right knee and lift your right foot behind you. Grasp the instep of the right foot with your right hand. Your knee should be pointing down to the floor. Keep your knees as close together as possible. Hold on to something with your left hand if necessary for steadiness. Change to the other side. Repeat twice on each side.

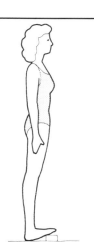

For calves

With your arms by your sides, stand upright on the balls of your feet on the edge of a step, book or brick so that your heels protrude backwards over the edge. Lower your heels until you feel the stretch in the back of your calves. Hold for 20 seconds. Hold on to a wall or chair to steady yourself if necessary.

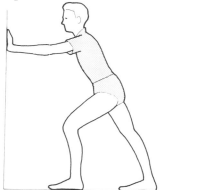

For calves

Stand in front of a wall. Take one step forward and push against the wall with your hands, arms straight. Flex forward knee and keep rear leg fully stretched, feet pointing forward, heels flat on floor. Lean forward until you feel a continuous stretch in the rear calf. Hold for 30 seconds (building to 60 seconds). Repeat with the other leg. Do this again with rear leg bent at the knee (for lower calf muscles). Repeat once for a few sessions, then twice.

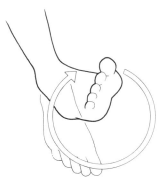

For ankles

Stand on your left foot or sit down on a chair and raise your right foot out in front of you. Rotate the foot at the ankle, ten times in each direction. Change to the other foot.

STRENGTHENING EXERCISES

Ideally, these exercises should be included after the warm-up and stretching exercises. They develop muscle strength and conditioning and are an essential part of a well-rounded exercise programme. They can also be included in circuit-training or in a programme using free weights or machine weights (like Nautilus, etc). Apart from maintaining muscle strength and endurance so that weakness and a decline in function are avoided, these exercises help to maintain muscle tone and produce an attractive body shape. Perhaps, most importantly, they have a beneficial effect on bone density, thickness and strength, so they help to alleviate the bone-loss that causes fractures with ageing.

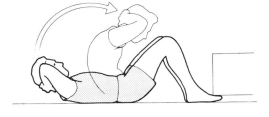

For more advanced sit-ups, lie on your back, knees bent, feet tucked under sofa, hands clasped behind head. With chin tucked in on chest, curl trunk to upright position, hold for count of one and slowly uncurl to starting position. Repeat 15 times, building up to 20.

Beginners press-up

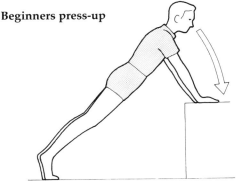

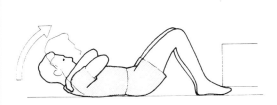

For hips and abdomen (sit-ups)

This one is for beginners. Lie on your back, knees bent, feet tucked under the sofa, hands on chest. With chin on chest, curl up, raising shoulders approximately 18 inches off the floor. Hold for a count of one and slowly lower to starting position. Repeat 10 times, building up to 20.

For chest, shoulders and backs of arms (press-ups)

Support the trunk with straight arms resting on flat hands on a table top, or something similar, with your body leaning forward at an angle of about 45 degrees to the vertical in a straight line. By bending the elbows, lower the body until the chest touches or is close to the table, then straighten the arms again. Repeat 10 times working up to 20. This is an easier version of the complete press-up (see page 106).

More advanced press-up

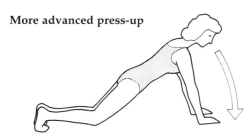

Lie face down with hands flat on the floor, shoulder width apart. Keeping the knees on the floor, push up until the arms are straight. Repeat 10 times, building up to 20.

Complete press-up

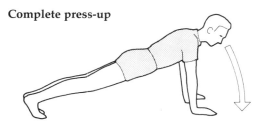

Lie face down with hands flat on the floor, shoulder width apart. Keeping your body straight, push up off the floor until the arms are straight. Lower chest to floor. Repeat 20 times, building up to 30.

For arms

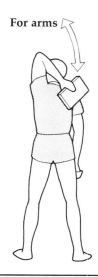

Stand upright with feet apart. In your left hand hold a dumbbell or a book or sand bag weighing about 3–5 pounds. Raise your left arm so that it is straight above your head. Bend the left elbow keeping the upper arm vertical until the hand holding the weight is at neck level behind your neck. Then straighten your arm so that it is vertical again. Repeat 10 times. Change to the other arm.

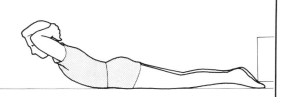

For lower back

Lie face down on the floor with your feet tucked under a chair or sofa, and your hands clasped behind your neck. Raise your head and trunk, hold for 5 seconds and lower. Repeat 10 times.

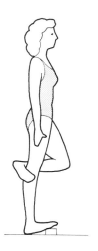

For calves

With your arms by your sides, stand upright on the ball of your right foot on the edge of a step, book or brick so that your heel protrudes backwards over the edge. Wrap the left foot round the back of the right knee. Raise yourself onto the ball of your foot and then down again so that the heel is lower than horizontal. Repeat 10 times. Change to the other foot. You may need to hold on to a chair or wall to steady yourself.

How much, how long and how often

Experts maintain that the risk of coronary heart disease can be substantially reduced by a regular programme of aerobic exercise consisting of three to five sessions per week, of 20–30 minutes duration, at an intensity that elicits a heart rate within 60–85% of the individual's maximum.

> 60% of maximum heart rate is found by subtracting your age from 220 and multiplying by $^{60}/_{100}$:
>
> e.g. for a person of 40, 60% maximum heart rate equals $220 - 40 = 180 \times {}^{60}/_{100} = 108$ beats per minute.
>
> 85% maximum heart rate in a 40 year old equals $180 \times {}^{85}/_{100} = 153$ beats per minute.

An ideal exercise programme would be one that includes the following four main components:

* warm-up/stretching

* muscle conditioning

* aerobic exercise

* warm-down/stretching

Table 11 gives a suggested exercise routine with recommended time spent on each element in a programme lasting thirty-five minutes or more.

HEART CONDITIONING AND WEIGHT CONTROL

If the goal in exercising is the development of cardio-respiratory endurance and weight reduction/control, the important factor in the training programme is the *total* energy used. To achieve these particular goals you need to aim for an energy expenditure of 1500–2000 Kcals per week. Table 12 gives the frequency, intensity, duration and type of training needed to achieve this level of energy expenditure (page 109). Table 14 gives the energy expenditure in Kcals per minute for a variety of activities (page 112).

HOW HARD ARE YOU EXERCISING?

One way of assessing how hard you are working is to take your pulse. Read the boxed paragraph on page 110 to discover how easy it is to take your pulse. However, many people find taking their pulse is a nuisance and just don't bother. Before we knew about maximum heart rate, oxygen consumption and energy expenditure, people would ease up or stop exerting themselves when they became too tired, too hot, or too out of breath, without analysing whether or not they should do so. Some researchers believe that utilizing our natural ability to estimate our levels of exertion for ourselves in this way is more reasonable than pulse-taking. They have used this natural 'knowing' as the basis for *perceived exertion scales* which relate the way a person feels at different levels of exercise intensity to the physiological changes that occur when exercising at those intensities.

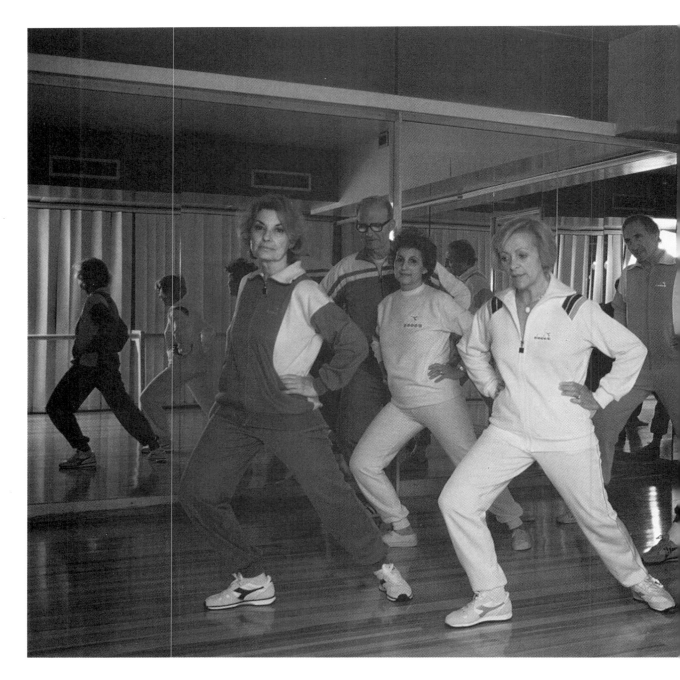

Table II Suggested exercise programme

	Activities	Recommended time
Warm-up	Walking/slow jogging and stretching exercises	10 minutes
Muscle conditioning	Muscle-strengthening exercises, weight-training with free weights or machine weights	5+ minutes
Aerobics	Fast walking, jogging, running, swimming, cycling, vigorous games, dancing, stair-climbing – continuous exercise	20+ minutes
Warm-down	Stretching exercises	5+ minutes
	Relaxation	2+ minutes

Source: Adapted from *Exercise in Health and Disease,* Pollock and Wilmore, W.B. Saunders (1990).

Table 12
Recommendations for using up the required amount of energy for heart conditioning and weight control

1. Frequency	3–5 days per week
2. Intensity	60–90% of maximum heart rate, i.e., 50–85% of maximum oxygen uptake
3. Duration	20–60 minutes (continuous)
4. Activity	Walking/running/jogging, cycling, dancing, rope-skipping, rowing, stair-climbing, swimming, skating
5. Weight training	8–10 exercises (8 to 12 repetitions of each) that condition the major muscle groups at least 2 days per week

(Adapted from the American College of Sports Medicine: Position statement on the recommended quantity and quality of exercise for developing and maintaining fitness in healthy adults. *Med. Sci. Sports* 10:vii-x, 1978. Revised and published in *Med. Sci. Sport Exerc.* in 1990).

Source: *Exercise in Health and Disease,* Pollock and Wilmore, W.B. Saunders (1990).

HOW TO TAKE A PULSE

1. Find your pulse while you are still exercising. If you are right-handed, place the middle three fingers of your right hand over the radial pulse on the thumb side of your left wrist (palm facing up), or over the left carotid artery in your neck below your earlobe near the angle of the jaw. Use your left hand if you are left-handed.

2. Stop exercising at a time that allows you to start counting immediately. Make certain the second hand on your watch is approaching a convenient setting before stopping.

3. Count your pulse for ten seconds, and then multiply this number by six to determine your heart rate in beats per minute (see page 107).

Source: *The Physician and Sportsmedicine.*

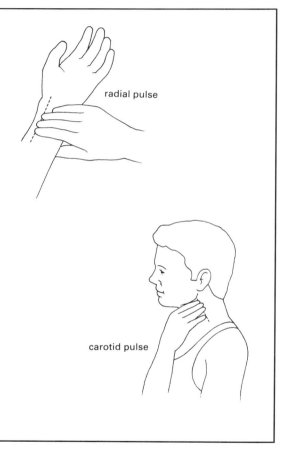

radial pulse

carotid pulse

The Borg Scale consists of fifteen Ratings of Perceived Exertion (RPE) that correspond to various heart rates (see Table 13, Borg perceived exertion scale with corresponding heart rates). As a measurement tool, the Borg Scale is simple, easy to learn to use, highly reliable and very accurate. It seems that everyone has the natural ability to assess accurately the intensity of the exercise in which they are engaged, simply by being aware of how they feel.

RPE could also be an effective measurement tool in assessing the intensity of exercise in everyday activities and may be a way of encouraging sedentary people to get into the habit of exercise. The idea is that you learn to identify the feeling of hard work that stops well short of exhaustion. Whether you are digging the garden, raking the leaves, or cleaning the car, this is a more natural way to determine energy output than to stop and take your pulse.

Table 13
Fifteen-point Borg perceived exertion scale with corresponding heart rates*

Rating of Perceived Exertion	Level of Exertion	Heart Rate Beats per min
6	Very, very light	60
7		70
8	Very light	80
9		90
10	Fairly light	100
11		110
12	Somewhat hard	120
13		130
14	Hard	140
15		150
16	Very hard	160
17		170
18	Very, very hard	180
19		190
20		200

*Rating of Perceived Exertion (RPE) × 10 = heart rate

Choice of exercise

Your choice of exercise, physical activity or sport will depend upon your aims, your state of physical fitness, your preferences and accessibility of facilities. Table 14 (page 112) shows a comparison of a number of alternatives with their strong and weak points.

It does not take an enormous amount of exercise to obtain considerable health benefits. A moderate amount of exercise, such as a daily two-mile walk, can produce significant improvements in health, including a lower mortality rate, when compared with more sedentary individuals. It is believed that covering ten miles a week, whether those miles are covered with brisk walking, jogging or cycling, will provide the same health benefits. Let's look at a few forms of exercise more closely.

WALKING

The benefits of walking are grossly underestimated. To maintain fitness it is as good as any aerobic activity if you walk sufficiently intensely. The body cannot tell whether you are swimming, running, cycling or walking. It is also an excellent way to lose fat weight. To realize these benefits, it is recommended to walk 20–30 minutes per day, four or five days a week at an intensity of 3.5–4 mph. In other words, you cover one mile in about 15–17 minutes.

If you have been sedentary, walking is the best exercise with which to start to improve your fitness. It has many advantages; it is cheap, accessible and safe. It does not require any special skill training and can be done in groups or families of people from the age of one upwards. It has a low risk of injury compared with running, in which the primary cause of injury is the force of impact when the feet hit the ground, a force equal to 2.5–3 times the body weight at each and every stride.

Table 14 Energy cost of various activities with their contributions to aspects of fitness (marked out of 7)

Remember for the risk of injury, the higher the score the greater the risk. For all the others, the higher the score the better. Energy costs are based on individuals weighing 56–80 kilos.

Activity	Energy Cost kilocalories/ min	Aerobic Stamina/ Cardiovascular Health	Local Muscle Endurance (anaerobic fitness)	Strength	Flexibility	Weight Control
Badminton	5–8	●●●– ●●●●	●●●●●	●●	●●●●	●●●
Canoeing	2.5–8	●●– ●●●●	●●●●●	●●●●● (upper body)	●●●	●●●●
Circuit training	10–14	●●●●●●●	●●●●●●	●●●●●●	●●●●●	●●●●●●●
Cricket: batting bowling	4.6–6.6 5.0–7.2	●●● ●●●●	●● ●●●●	●●●● ●●●●	●●●● ●●●●	●●● ●●●●
Cycling: 5.5mph 9.4mph	3.6–5.1 5.6–8.0	●●●● ●●●●●●	●●●	●● ●●	●● ●●	●●●● ●●●●●●
Dancing: aerobic	6–9	●●●●●– ●●●●●●	●●●●● ●●●●	●●	●●●●●– ●●●●●●	●●●●●
Gardening: digging/ mowing/raking	6–10	●●●– ●●●●	●– ●●●●	●●●– ●●●●	●●	●●●●
Golf	4.8–8.8	●●●– ●●●●● (in older age groups)	●●	●●	●●●	●●●●
Hockey	6–12	●●●● ●●●●●●	●●●●●●	●●●●	●●●●	●●●●●
Horse riding	3.7–10	●●– ●●●●●	●●●●	●●●	●●	●●
Jogging/Running 11min 30sec/mile 9min/mile 8min/mile 7min/mile	7.6–11.0 10.8–15.4 11.9–16.5 13.3–18.0	●●●– ●●●●●●●	●●– ●●●●●	●●	●●	●●●●●●●
Rowing	8–14	●●●●●– ●●●●●●●	●●●●●●●	●●●●●– ●●●●●●●	●●●	●●●●●●
Rugby	6–12	●●●●– ●●●●●●	●●●●●●	●●●– ●●●●●●	●●●●●	●●●●
Sailing	2.5–6	●●– ●●●	●●●●●– ●●●●●●	●●●●●	●●●●	●●
Skiing: downhill	5.5–9	●●●●	●●●●– ●●●●●●	●●●●●	●●●●●	●●●●
cross country	8–11.5	●●●●●●●	●●●– ●●●●	●●●●	●●●●	●●●●●●●
Soccer	6–12	●●●●– ●●●●●	●●●●●●	●●●●	●●●– ●●●●	●●●●●
Squash	10–15	●●●●●– ●●●●●●●	●●●●●●●	●●●	●●●●●	●●●●●
Swimming: backstroke breaststroke crawl – fast crawl – slow	9.5–13.5 9.1–13.0 8.7–12.5 7.2–10.2	●●●●– ●●●●●●●	●●●●– ●●●●●●	●●●●	●●●●●	●●●●●
Tennis	6–9	●●●– ●●●●	●●	●●●	●●●●	●●●●
Walking: 3.5mph	3.5–5.0	●●●●●	●●●	●●	●●	●●●●
Weight training	3–8	●●●●	●●●●●	●●●●●●●	●	●●●

Example of a week's activities with an energy cost of approximately 2000 kilocalories for an individual weighing 70 kilos

* Alternatively use the exercise bike for 5 × 12 mins, or walk the dog for 25 mins a day.

Walking	— 3 × 30 mins at 3.5 mph	= 400 kilocalories
*Gardening	— 1 hour including digging, mowing, raking leaves etc	= 500 kilocalories
Squash	— 45 minutes	= 540 kilocalories
Swimming	— 2 × 30 mins	= 480 kilocalories
	TOTAL	1920 kilocalories

~ity	Body Shape	Bone Health	Risk of Injury	Convenience Access/Facilities	Skill Acquisition	Competition	Sociability
~ninton	•••	•••	•••	••	•••••	•••••••	•••••••
~oeing	••••	•••	•••	•	••••	••••	•••••••
~uit training	•••••••	•••••	••••	••	•••	••	•
~ket: batting	•••	••••	••••••	••	•••••••	•••••••	•••••••
bowling	••••	••••	••••	••	•••••••	•••••••	•••••••
~ing: 5.5mph	•••	••					
9.4mph	•••	••	•••••• (if on road)	••••••	••	••	••
~cing: aerobic	•••••	[1] •••••• [2] ••	••••• ••	•• ••	•• ••	• •	••••• •••••
~dening: digging/ ~owing/raking	•••	••	••	•••••••	•	•	•
~f	•••	••	••	•	•••••••	•••••••	•••••••
~key	••••	••••••– •••••••	••••••	••	•••••••	•••••••	•••••••
~se riding	••	••••	••••••	•	•••••••	•••	•••••
~ing/Running ~in 30sec/mile ~/mile ~/mile	•••	•••••••	•••••	•••••••	••	••	•– •••••
~ing	•••••	•••••– ••••••	•••	•	••••	•••••••	•••••••
~by	••••	••••••	•••••••	•••	•••••••	•••••••	•••••••
~ng	••	••••	•••	•	•••••	•••••••	•••••••
~ng: downhill	•••	••••	•••••••	•	•••••••	•••	••••
cross country	••••••	••••	•••	•	••••	•	••••
~er	••••	••••••	••••••	•••	•••••••	•••••••	•••••••
~ash	••••	••••	••••••	•	•••••••	•••••••	•••••••
~mming: backstroke breaststroke crawl – fast crawl – slow	••••	•••	•	•	••••	•	•
~nis	••••	••••	•••	••	•••••••	•••••••	•••••••
~king: 3.5mph	•••	•••	•	•••••••	•	•	•– •••••••
~ght training	••••••	••••••	••••	••	•••	••	••

[1] High impact   [2] Low impact

GOLF

Walking golf courses is an excellent form of exercise of moderate intensity. A study of golfers playing three times a week on an 18-hole course, where the estimated distance walked per round was 8000 yards, showed that the average calorie expenditure of walking the course was 470 Kcal; the average weight lost by the golfers over a period of four months on this programme was 3.5 lbs, and the blood cholesterol levels showed a significant improvement. Since it is accepted that the protective effect of leisure-time physical activity with respect to the risk of coronary heart disease occurs through mechanisms involving favourable changes in blood cholesterol and other fats, this study shows that golfers who play three times a week and who walk *briskly* round the course, are doing enough physical exercise to improve significantly their chances of avoiding a heart attack. It is also true that, since golf is a leisure-time activity and not simply an exercise programme, regular participation by players tends to be fairly consistent.

AEROBICS

Low-impact aerobics involves exercising to music while always keeping one foot in contact with the floor.

By contrast, high-impact aerobics involves hopping and jumping movements followed by a forceful landing on the foot (see Table 15). Low-impact aerobics is less strenuous and safer than high-impact aerobics, because it places less stress on the joints. This kind of exercise is preferable for people when they are first starting an exercise programme or if they are overweight, and/or getting on in years; the injury rate in low-impact aerobics is considerably lower. Low-impact aerobics has been criticized for not being of sufficient intensity to develop cardiovascular fitness. In fact, you can achieve the same amount of work with a low-intensity exercise as with one of high intensity if you perform the former for a longer period of time. Again, like the golfers walking the golf courses three times a week, these data on low-impact aerobics suggest that activity of *any* type improves health even when fitness measures, such as maximum oxygen consumption, do not change substantially. Regular physical activity of moderate intensity is linked to lower rates of chronic disease and to an increased life-span. However, while high-intensity/low-volume work is related to cardiovascular (heart) fitness, low-intensity/high-volume work is more useful for burning calories and for weight loss.

EXERCISE FOR BONE HEALTH

A decrease in bone density gradually occurs in both sexes from the age of about thirty-five to forty onwards. In post-menopausal women, this bone-loss is accelerated and there is an increased risk of osteoporosis and bone fractures.

Since weight-bearing physical activity is essential for bone health, exercise can play a direct role in maintaining bone health throughout the mature adult years and can attenuate the loss of bone in women after the menopause. The question is: what kind of exercise is needed to do this job? Aerobic activities to improve cardiovascular fitness

Table 15

High- and low-impact aerobic activities

High impact	Low impact
Jogging/running	Walking
Basket/volleyball	Cycling
Hopping/jumping	Swimming
Rope-skipping	Rowing
Aerobic dancing (high impact)	Stair-climbing
	Aerobic dancing (low impact)
Vigorous games	

Source: Pollock, 'Exercise prescription for the elderly' in Eckert and Spirduso (eds), *Physical Activity and Aging*, Human Kinetics, Champaign, IL (1989).

required to hop as high as possible for a few seconds every morning and evening, whilst others were required to squeeze a tennis ball as hard as possible three times, morning and night. His results showed a considerable increase in bone density in the particular bones involved. The conclusion he reached was that it is bone-stressing that is important in improving bone density.

Risks associated with exercise

EXERCISE ADDICTION

Many people exercise far too little, but many others exercise far too much. How much is too much and why? Leisure-time exercisers who work out or run two to three hours a day to the detriment of their family life and work, and who will not stop even when injured and in pain, are almost certainly exercise addicts. If forced to stop for any reason, these exercise extremists can suffer from sleeplessness, restlessness, loss of appetite and depression – symptoms similar to those seen with drug withdrawal. In fact, these people may be addicted to the endorphins released by exercise – the so-called 'runner's high'.

INJURIES

Other people may exercise to excess because they believe that if exercise is a good thing, then more of it must be better. But excessive exercise increases the risk of injuries. Injuries can be avoided with adequate warm-up and warm-down exercises, and by not exercising

may have little or no effect on bone density although it should be kept in mind that *any* increase in physical activity may have a positive effect on bone mass in women who have been very sedentary. Nevertheless, swimming, walking (unless vigorous) and cycling, whilst excellent fitness-producing activities, are of questionable value in preventing bone-loss or rebuilding lost bone, as they do not involve substantial weight-bearing exercise. Activities that are recommended include running, jogging, weight-training, high-impact aerobics, stair-climbing, racket sports and dancing, all of which will have general skeletal benefits. But these benefits need to be weighed against the increased risk of injury in these kinds of activities.

Recently an orthopaedic surgeon has been prescribing tiny amounts of weight-bearing exercise designed to put stress on specific bones – for example, his patients have been

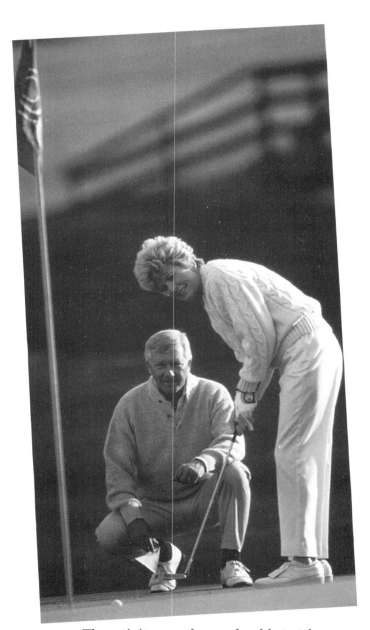

The activity you choose should stretch you physically, fit your lifestyle and, above all, be enjoyable

with a high temperature, when ill or under the weather. Also, proper equipment is essential – especially footwear in runners, walkers and hikers, helmets in cyclists, hard-hats in riders, and, if possible, protective glasses for squash.

MORTALITY RATE

If a person carries on exercising to extremes, despite injuries, it is likely that this person may need psychological help. Instead of prolonging life, he or she may actually be shortening it. A well-known study of Harvard alumni by American Professor Ralph Paffenbarger of Stanford University School of Medicine showed that whilst regular, moderate leisure-time exercise may prolong life, the mortality rate went up in those who exercised over a certain level (see page 120). The cut-off point was a weekly energy expenditure in physical activity greater than 3500 Kcal. According to Table 14 (showing the energy cost of a variety of types of exercise) this would be equal each week to 5–6 hours running, or 8 hours cycling.

Mae West may have had a point when she said 'too much of a good thing can be wonderful', but it doesn't seem to apply in the case of the compulsive exerciser.

STRESS AND THE IMMUNE SYSTEM

Exercise may enhance the immune response and ward off infection by regulating an assortment of hormones and other chemicals, released into the blood stream, that alleviate stress and improve the immune response. Conversely, however, acute, exhaustive exercise may create too much stress and damage the immune response. The level of exercise which may be damaging will depend on the individual and his or her state of health at any particular time. On a more positive note, it is possible that *moderate* exercise may slow down the usual decrease in immune response that is seen with ageing.

AIR POLLUTION

The air we breathe contains a number of pollutants of which carbon monoxide and ozone pose the greatest threat to exercisers.

The principal sources of carbon monoxide in the environment are car exhaust fumes and cigarette smoke. When carbon monoxide enters the blood, less oxygen can be transported and less is available to the muscles. The heart has to work harder and beat faster to deliver more blood to compensate for the lower oxygen available. Strenuous exercise in heavy traffic for thirty minutes can produce the same levels of carbon monoxide in the blood as smoking ten cigarettes. Seeking the shade of trees when exercising in the heat can also be detrimental as polluted air can remain trapped under the trees. Ozone is a predominant component of polluted city air that can cause obstruction of the airways after a few hours' exposure. Ozone levels increase considerably on bright, sunny days.

Exercisers can minimize their risk from air pollution with the following precautions: avoid exercising during peak traffic hours and when the sun is brightest and hottest in the middle of the day; exercise in open areas where air currents can move about freely, dispersing pollutants (but if you have to run or

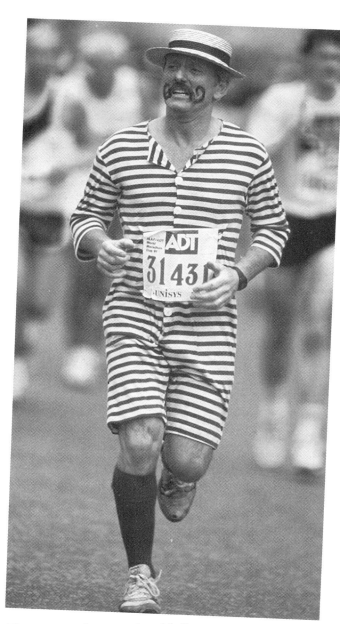

No reason why you shouldn't run a marathon – but you must train properly for it and check with your doctor first

117

walk on pavements, position yourself as far from the kerb as possible); never exercise in a road tunnel; avoid cigarette smoke, your own or other people's, before and after exercise.

EXERCISING IN THE HEAT

The principal concern when performing any kind of physical activity in the heat is dehydration. The best fluids to replace those lost are water and a dilute electrolyte solution (which contains salts of sodium and potassium, of the kind prescribed for severe diarrhoea). Sugary drinks are not as good, because they are not rapidly absorbed by the body. In addition, since salt is lost due to the increased rate of sweating in the heat, a little extra salt on the food is recommended (people with high blood pressure or those taking diuretics should consult their doctors before increasing their salt intake).

Warm-up, warm-down and injury prevention

Every exercise session should begin with a brief warm-up routine consisting of stretching exercises (see pages 100-104) to develop and maintain flexibility, and performed after a few minutes of walking or gentle jogging so that the heart rate, blood flow and breathing are all increased, preparing the body for more vigorous physical activity. Stretching the major muscle groups will also prevent injury due to muscle tears.

At the end of the exercise session, when the muscles, ligaments, tendons and other tissues surrounding the joints are warm, flexibility exercises should be done to increase the range of movements of the joints. When stretching and flexing, it is most important never to use a 'bouncing movement', but simply to hold the stretched or flexed position for about twenty seconds. Finally, an exercise session should finish off with a few minutes of total relaxation, lying if possible on the back and taking deep, abdominal breaths.

When to exercise

There seems to be a general consensus that the best time to exercise is in the early morning. This may be a rumour put about by the 'larks' amongst us who relish the idea of a run before breakfast; it does little to encourage the 'owls' who find it difficult to stand upright for the first hour or two after waking. Here is some good news for the 'owls'. For people who are in their middle lives or older, the worst time to exercise is first thing in the morning and up to two hours after rising. This is a favourite time for heart attacks to occur, because the heart muscle is particularly sensitive to exertion when a person first gets up in the morning.

Exercising before a meal can help in weight

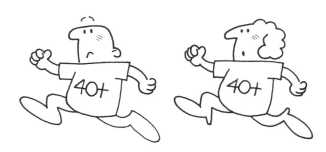

control if the exercise is sufficiently vigorous – achieving a heart rate of 60% of maximum or above (see page 107) – which raises the metabolic rate to produce an 'after burn' effect when the exercise stops. In other words, the body goes on using up calories at a higher rate than normal for several hours after exercising has stopped. Other advantages of taking vigorous exercise before meals are a blunting of the appetite and replacement of the body's carbohydrate stores by the starches and sugars in the meal without their being converted to fat.

On the other hand, exercising vigorously too soon *after* a meal is not advised because the large reservoir of blood that has flowed to the abdomen to help digestion and absorption of food is shunted away from the gastrointestinal tract and towards the working muscles in the limbs. Digestion is interrupted which can be extremely uncomfortable. But flopping on the nearest sofa after a meal is also a mistake. Courtiers in the eighteenth century had the right idea; they would take a gentle, pleasant walk in the garden after eating. Mild exercise like this at a level just high enough to keep the blood moving has two possible advantages:

1. To help the movement of food through the gut by speeding up the emptying of the stomach and relieving that full feeling.

2. To help in controlling or losing weight by boosting the 'thermic effect' of food which is the increase in the metabolic rate due to the energy needed for digestion. This thermic effect can double when gentle exercise is taken after a meal.

For 'exercise' read 'activity'

In this chapter I have explained the exercise needed for total fitness, a programme that incorporates exercise for stamina, strength and flexibility (see Tables 11 and 12). This is based on the 1990 recommendations of the American College of Sports Medicine (ACSM), for the quantity and quality of exercise needed to develop and maintain fitness in healthy adults. Particular emphasis has been placed on cardiovascular fitness.

In the USA, it has been realized by health specialists promoting exercise and fitness that these guidelines may actually be having the opposite effect to that intended, because they are discouraging the vast majority of people from doing anything at all. (Eighty-five per cent of Americans do not take any regular exercise.)

The question currently on the minds of the experts is whether fitness is necessary for health. Apart from cardiac patients who are rehabilitating, the majority of regular vigorous exercisers are doing it for reasons other than possible health benefits. My doctor, a self-confessed food addict, runs two miles a day because, with exercise, he 'feels better, can concentrate, keeps the weight off and enjoys sex more'. In other words, he has more energy for work and play, and life generally takes on a rosier hue. But he is one of only 6% of the adult population in this country who exercise regularly. Of the other 94%, no doubt some have a go, but the on-going, long-term participation in exercise fitness programmes is phenomenally low – I know, I am one of the recidivists! Fortunately for me and

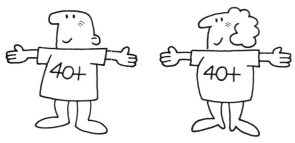

millions of others like me, moderate physical activity is the key to realizing major health benefits, in particular, to reducing the risk of heart disease. How do we know this? Forty years ago it was found that when the drivers of London double-decker buses were compared with the more physically active conductors, the latter had significantly less coronary heart disease than the bus drivers. Similarly, in San Francisco, longshoremen who were handling heavy cargo had a much lower incidence of fatal heart disease than men holding physically less demanding jobs. Postmen are protected against heart disease because they walk so much. Sitting here at my desk, it is patently obvious that many of us have jobs that require no more activity than pressing the word-processor keys. With mechanization and automation, the development of robots and computers, strenuous physical effort has been progressively eliminated from work. We, in the West, have become increasingly sedentary as a result. Nowadays, it is physical activity performed during leisure hours that may help reduce the risk of heart disease and other chronic conditions. A renowned study by Professor Jerry Morris of London University showed that desk-bound civil servants who regularly swam, played badminton, hill-walked, and

performed heavy jobs at home like digging and concreting, etc. had a significantly reduced incidence of heart attacks compared with office workers who had a sedentary lifestyle.

More recently, a study already mentioned, by Professor Ralph Paffenbarger (see page 116), has shown that the death rate from all causes was significantly reduced by 28% in people who put in enough weekly physical activity, like walking, climbing stairs and playing sports, to account for a weekly energy output of 2000 Kcal or more. Moreover, if the energy used on physical activities of this kind reached a weekly total of 3500 Kcal, the relative risk of death from any cause was less than half of that of the most sedentary subjects. At levels above 3500 Kcal, however, the trend reversed which implies that an optimal energy output in physical activity is about 3500 Kcal a week. (See Table 14, page 112, showing energy costs of various physical activities.) The target of 2000 Kcal-plus of physical activity a week could easily be achieved simply by increasing the amount of activity in your daily routine, e.g. walking instead of driving short distances, climbing the stairs instead of taking the lift, etc. Although some would argue that these moderate measures are not sufficiently aerobic or 'vigorous' to reduce the risk of coronary disease, the study looked at death rates from all causes. Since more people die from heart attacks than any other disease in developed countries, the 2000 Kcal levels of physical activity in the study, it is argued, must have a positive effect on the death rates from heart attacks.

Clinicians today are much more interested in their patient's activity patterns than in prescribing well-defined exercise programmes and many believe that the ACSM guidelines are unnecessarily strenuous for many people. While a certain level of physical fitness is related to good health, those that are very fit are not necessarily the most healthy. Running is a high intensity activity that increases cardiovascular endurance, uses up a lot of calories and helps control weight, but it carries with it a high incidence of injuries and is certainly not to be recommended for everyone. In any case, a lot of people – and I am one – hate running. What is important is to find a physical activity pattern that fits your life, *stretches* you a little past your usual limit, and is a *pleasure*. As one eminent specialist said, 'You don't have to go out and kill yourself to improve your health, just get out there and enjoy life.'

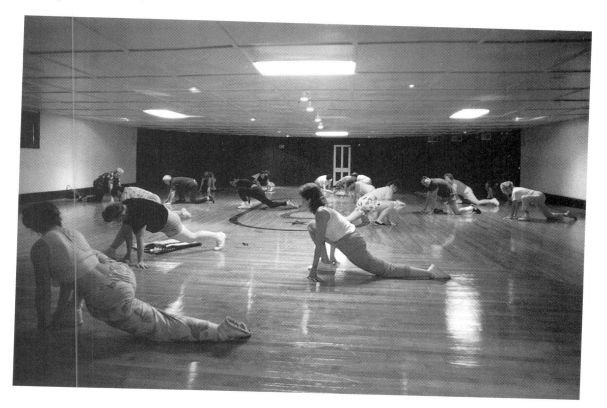

How Other People Exercise

What happens to top athletes after they've passed their peak and gone beyond the forty-year marker? Some, certainly, strive to maintain their fitness and health, and it would be beneficial to see how some of them go about it.

Lynn Davies

Lynn and I met in the early 1980s, when we both competed in the TV 'Superstars' series. We ran, jumped and played against each other on about five occasions.

It must be said that Lynn is not like other forty-seven-year-olds. Not because he long-jumped 26 ft 6 ins to an Olympic Gold medal in Tokyo in 1972 or because he enjoyed and enjoys training and exercise, but because he is an exceptionally gifted athlete and will be till he trickles down the sink.

In one sense he is not a good role model since, in spite of his unassuming modesty, he started off with several advantages. He has always been highly co-ordinated (hand, eye, foot), and a talented ball player and gymnast.

Natural talent is by itself the foundation for success in most sports but by itself it is not enough. The desire or the need to achieve, based on whatever reason, must accompany that talent. In Lynn's case not only is he naturally talented, but he had a need for success and, luckily for him, he enjoyed the work necessary to achieve that success.

It is this enjoyment that keeps Lynn running now at the age of forty-seven and has probably helped him cope with the ageing process. In one way Lynn is a terrific role model in that it must be much harder for a Gold-medal athlete to come to terms with

physically changing circumstances than someone who hasn't known that level of physical commitment and degree of success.

Lynn's exercise regime has always been an important part of his life. In his early twenties at Cardiff College, in addition to his physical education studies, he was also under the guidance of Ron Pickering, undertaking punishing speed-track sessions and heavy

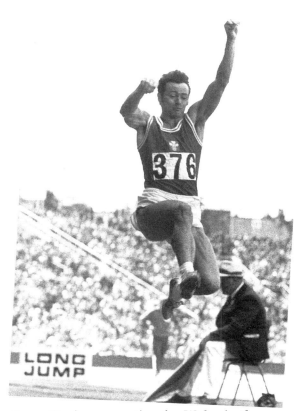

Lynn Davies competing for Wales in the British Commonwealth Games, 1970

weight-training, to enhance and develop the skills required for long-jumping. It paid off; besides winning the Gold Medal at Tokyo, he also competed in the 1968 Mexico and 1976 Munich Olympics.

Lynn's current exercise routine

Lynn is a fund of knowledge about training and he prefaced an outline of his current programme with these two tips:

* it's not the intensity, it's the consistency of training that is most important

* you need the desire to do it and you need to enjoy whatever form of training you undertake, if you intend to continue training in the long term

In spite of a heavy regime of training throughout his life Lynn is lucky in that, although weaknesses in his knees and Achilles' tendon limit his interest in running long distances, he is in excellent physiological shape. This allows him to take some form of exercise every day. His regime is based around running just over two miles a day (15–20 minutes) or about five miles on a mountain bike (20 minutes) and light weight-training.

He does nothing competitively other than recreational tennis or squash against some of his colleagues at BBC Wales in Cardiff. Lynn has never smoked and drinks modestly but has paid little attention to his diet, suggesting that training allows you the scope to enjoy your vices. I presume he means meat, lots of dairy products and lashings of ginger beer.

Chris Ralston

Chris Ralston and I have been pals for the last twenty years. Undoubtedly the greatest debt I have to rugby is the friends I made through the game. Hackneyed cliché it may be, but making friends is one of the great side benefits of team games.

Chris played club rugby for Richmond for about twenty years and also represented Middlesex, the Barbarians, England and the British Lions. He was a second-row forward and the combination of him, Roger Uttley and myself was often unkindly referred to as a likely source of extras for any of the films from the Hammer House of Horror school of cinema (no make-up required). I must say, in our collective defence, that we all felt we had graduated from the Marlboro man on horseback school of rugged charm.

So this is Chris's health 'n exercise story. Chris is forty-six, 6 ft 6 ins and weighs in at 250 lbs. He has smoked heavily in his time, but hasn't smoked for two years. He drinks, but at the time of writing was on a two-month break. His diet, without him making a big deal of it, is, and has been, increasingly health-aware – sugar-free, Flora, mineral water, skimmed milk, brown bread; he likes vegetarian food but still eats meat.

Like all big and/or heavy men, who play sport, particularly physical-contact games, Chris has paid the price as he's grown older. His knee joints and, more recently, his hips have suffered, to the extent that at forty-five he had to have a hip-replacement operation. This has limited the exercise options available to him.

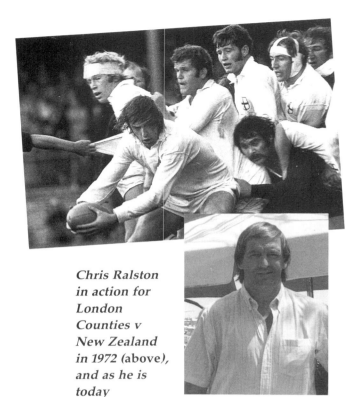

Chris Ralston in action for London Counties v New Zealand in 1972 (above), and as he is today

Chris's exercise routine, past and present

Up until the age of eighteen, Chris participated in most types of sport and, because of his size and ball-handling ability, was particularly successful at rugby. Never noted for his training appetite, he always looked after himself; club training two nights a week during the season and two three-mile runs (20 minutes) a week formed the basis of his exercise.

In his mid-thirties, because he was living and working in central London, he used health clubs. As his knees continued to give him trouble he has increasingly used this type of facility, specifically taking advantage of their aerobic and circuit-training classes. He has also used the weight-supporting exercise machines such as the stairmaster, the rower and the lifecycle.

His hip operation has made him increasingly aware that health and mobility cannot be taken for granted and you need to work at them in the way that's most beneficial for you. He now works out in a local gym for an hour or so a day, doing different routines on different days and mixing the weight-supporting cardiovascular machines with circuit-training classes.

His diet, nutrition and alcohol consumption reflect his increased health awareness. He has reduced a mid-thirties' cigarette consumption of up to fifty a day down to none; that is an indication of the dedication and concern he is now showing to alter his life. It's not everyone's choice of route but it seems to work for Chris.

Rachael Heyhoe Flint

For twenty-four years, until 1984, Rachael played cricket for England. She was capped fifty-one times in Test and One-Day Internationals. She was captain for eleven years, during which time England astonishingly never lost a Test match. This ran alongside being goalkeeper for the Staffordshire (twenty-five years) and England hockey teams and being a county squash player. On retiring from playing at the age of forty-three she took up golf and now plays off five. Rachael had the benefit of having not only outstanding hand-eye co-ordination and talented parents (both PE teachers), but also a ruthless streak, cunningly hidden under the most modest, laid-back, laughing personality.

Rachael is fifty-one, weighs 142 lbs and has to be aware of what she eats so she can drink 'more than a lady is meant to'. She eats no butter, sweets, dessert, sugar or potatoes and prefers chicken, fish or pasta to red meat. Her diet is a function of both taste and health awareness. She used to smoke about ten cigarettes a day before she was married but gave it up about twenty years ago when she realized how harmful it was. She now feels she has an obsession about smoking and the dangers of passive smoking. She enjoys wine with meals; her preferred drinks are chilled dry cider and a brandy or three as a nightcap. Having been in a team sport environment Rachael is a social drinker, but is aware of her obligations to her own well-being.

Rachael's current exercise routine

After Dartford Physical Education College, Rachael played squash, cricket, hockey, netball, lacrosse and tennis.

Since 1977, she has jogged most mornings about a mile with the dog. It's now just an extension to her daily routine. She works at a golf hotel and leisure centre which has a gym and a pool, but is forever failing to take advantage of the facilities. She plays little squash but a lot of golf, the appeal being not only the competitive challenge but also the company of people she plays with. Rachael seems to me to have got it all well worked out.

Right: *Rachael Heyhoe Flint swapped cricket for golf*

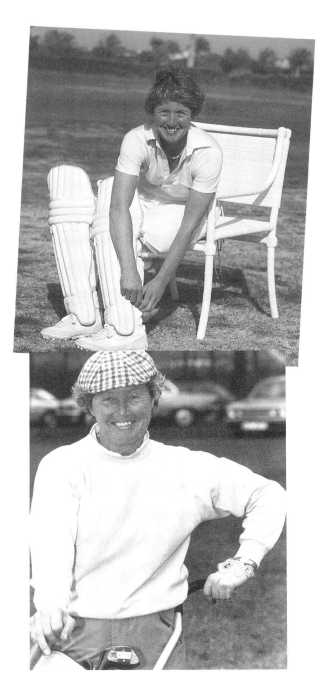

125

Brough Scott

Brough may have a unique educational background for a professional jump jockey (Radley and Oxford) and an unusual Christian name, and much more than an athlete's ability to express himself. But he is absolutely typical in that he has that one preoccupation of all jockeys and probably even ex-jockeys: weight.

At forty-eight, and 5 ft 8 ins, he weighs in at 150 lbs, just a few pounds heavier than when he rode some twenty to twenty-five years ago. 'Anyone can get thin and lose weight; saunas, lime juice and no food does the trick. But you need physical strength and mental stamina to control a horse.' The inference is that strength doesn't come from a bottle of Rose's Lime Cordial. The balancing equation for jockeys would seem to be a lightness in the saddle without a sacrifice of strength to control and dominate, if necessary, the mount and the other riders.

Surprisingly, Brough's current diet, even though once he, as a jockey, may have been obsessed with food, seems quite normal. Taste, rather than health or diet, appears to dictate what he eats. He has a preference for fish rather than red meat, cuts out the heart-stopper breakfast fry-up and steers clear of a morning egg. Nothing too unusual in that.

Brough drinks socially; wine with meals, the occasional beer, but little or no spirits. This Lent, however, he gave up alcohol, in the same way and probably for the same reasons that some people regularly give up drinking for a month each year (usually February!).

He no longer smokes, having given it up (twenty a day) after university, when he made

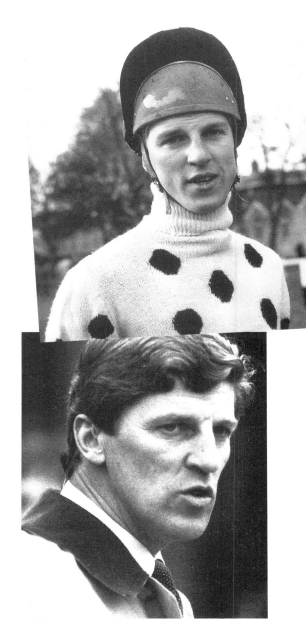

Brough Scott, professional jockey and professional commentator

a conscious decision to become a jump jockey. Perceiving himself as not being the best jockey in the world and realizing that, as an amateur, he needed all the help he could get, giving up smoking was a small part of the process. He hasn't smoked since. A few years ago he had a viral infection which manifested itself as a sharp pain in the chest. His discomfort was not eased by the fact that he was on a plane and had to be carried off. All of which puts one's own mortality into focus, so that even giving up cigars is an easier decision to make.

Brough had eight full seasons in the sport, four as an amateur and four as a professional. One of his proudest moments, a year after turning professional, was, with a plate in his arm, winning The Imperial Cup at Sandown.

Brough's current exercise routine

Even if he is an enthusiastic and successful player of games at school, a man who, post-puberty, seems cut out to be a jockey (unless he is extremely gifted in other areas) wouldn't have the weight or build to be anything other than a distance runner or a ski jumper. I don't think Brough had the inclination or opportunity for those two sports. He was twenty-one before he launched himself into riding, having got involved with a local trainer at the age of fifteen. I'm given to understand that a jockey's life is haphazard, that you're on your own and you get fit by race riding. If you can exist that way, have determination, keep your weight low but maintain sufficient strength, have talent and are invited to ride the best mounts, I think you get to be called Lester.

Now, Brough, father of four, sees himself as being fit and has obviously, like all athletes, learnt to live with his body as an instrument. However, when I asked him what he does now for exercise, it was apparent that he does little in the way of a formalized training routine. Perhaps he runs once in a blue moon, a little recreational tennis and he did once run the London Marathon. However, Brough feels it's not necessary for him to swim, run, cycle, etc. because he has a couple of five-year-old horses he cares for. He gets up early to go and feed, water and muck them out and rides for about an hour twice a week. His job as an interviewer, presenter and editor involves much walking, standing around and travelling and he sees that as just as good a way of taking exercise as the more ritualized way I prefer. For Brough, it's his route.

Roger Uttley

Roger has a distinguished sporting pedigree, both as a player and a communicator. He was coach to the England 1991 World Cup and Grand Slam teams, played in the previous England Grand Slam team (1980) and was a member of the undefeated 1974 British Lions team. Some record; and it spans two decades.

Now aged forty-one, weighing 229 lbs and at 6 ft 4 ins, Roger has always been a 'big lad, daft about sport'. At the age of about fifteen his main interest was cycling, ''cos I was good at it'. He also has an awareness that, to do well, you need to put in the groundwork. There is no substitute for getting in the miles.

So, at eighteen his size may have precluded

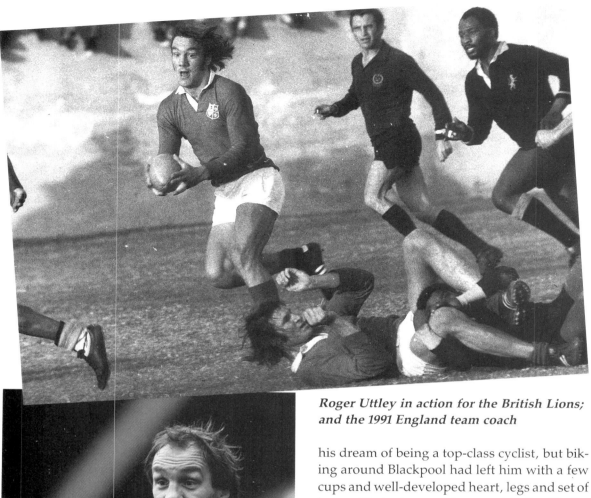

Roger Uttley in action for the British Lions; and the 1991 England team coach

his dream of being a top-class cyclist, but biking around Blackpool had left him with a few cups and well-developed heart, legs and set of lungs. He took up rugby, went to the Northumberland College of Education, joined Gosforth Rugby Club at the same time as Jack Rowle, Peter Dixon and David Robinson, and the rest, as they say, is hysteria.

Actually it wasn't hysteria, it was fifteen years of tremendous enjoyment, earned, however, in a collision sport which inflicted physical and lasting damage. Roger's career may look good on paper but on X-ray the legacy isn't quite so impressive. Back pain, referred stresses and strains and periods of hospitalization meant that, in 1981, the enjoyment of playing no longer outweighed the postmatch pain – and so he retired.

Roger's current exercise routine

Roger's diet has not changed much over the years: regular meals with a preference for granary bread and skimmed milk. He is now, for reasons of taste rather than health, eating less red meat. His alcohol consumption has always been modest. He doesn't drink at home unless he's got friends round; he'll have wine with a meal, a social beer at weekends and no spirits. Roger, surprisingly, does have the occasional cigarette, although, I've noticed, they're usually other people's.

'Chris, my wife, thinks I'm obsessive about exercise. Maybe she's right; I have a need – vanity perhaps – but unless I exercise I don't feel a complete person.

'When I stopped playing it took a long time to feel right, but I carried on with a limited exercise routine which was, of course, without the weekly physical setbacks of a game. I could have chosen to give it all away and watch TV but I didn't; I kept to a simple routine, even on a cold Tuesday night when it was raining. It came right.'

Roger is Head of Physical Training at Harrow School; this gives him an opportunity denied to most of us to indulge in his passion for exercise, competition and sport. His office is ten feet from an indoor pool and surrounded by playing fields. Purgatory if you don't like games but like Heaven if you do.

Roger will work out every day. He either swims 800 metres freestyle (about 14 minutes) or runs three miles (18–21 minutes). He plays tennis, golf and basketball. Currently he is, in his age group, world-ranked 7th on the ergo rowing machine over 2500 metres (8.06).

Naomi James

Dame Naomi James and I met as contestants on an episode of the 'Krypton Factor', alongside Richard Fox (king of slalom canoeists) and Beryl Burton (queen of cycling).

In 1977–78 Naomi single-handedly circumnavigated the globe. That's easy to write but a lot more difficult to do; you can read all about it in her book (*At One with the Sea*). She also competed in the 1980 single-handed Transatlantic race and won the 1982 Round Britain and Ireland race in a trimaran. In 1983 she gave birth to Lois and stopped sailing. Born in New Zealand, Naomi now lives in Paris with her Canadian husband Eric.

Naomi is forty-two, weighs about 140 lbs and has done so since her late teens; she is 5 ft 8 ins tall. Her diet is health-aware without being obsessive. She has become more nutrition-conscious, in part through trying to teach Lois (eight), good eating habits. So it's don't cram your body with fats and cut down on salt; fish and white meat in preference to red meat, and awareness of the benefits of fibre and less sugar. 'Good eating habits should be inculcated at an early age.' She enjoys wine with a meal but doesn't drink spirits. Naomi gave up smoking in 1974, having had a fifteen-a-day habit. She hasn't smoked since and found it quite easy to stop, 'because it's such a half-witted thing to do'.

Naomi's current exercise routine

Naomi's exercise routine has always been opportunity- and activity-based. In fact she probably wouldn't think of it as anything so

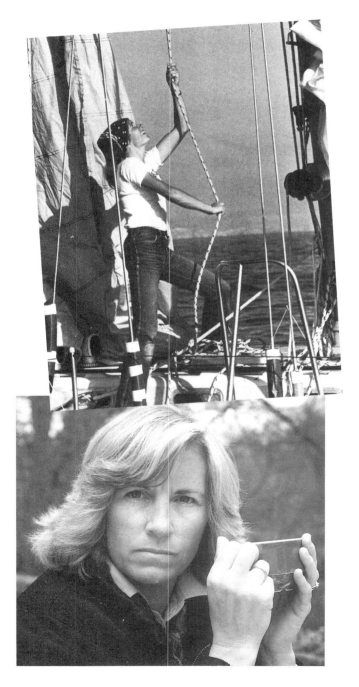

grand as an exercise routine.

Growing up in New Zealand, her teenage years were based around showing, training and riding horses. Ritualized sport, such as I enjoy, was not Naomi's path or inclination.

She married world-renowned yachtsman Rob James and had the opportunity to sail, which she did. I don't know much about single-handed sailing but I suspect it means pulling and lifting, and getting up and stretching, and boredom and fear, and an escape-route and not an escape-route, and a prison and achievement and joy, and expensive and a way of trying to establish one's worth, and lots and lots of activity in a confined space. But what do I know?

Naomi then lived in Gloucestershire and played some tennis till she hurt her shoulder skiing and then took to golf. She enjoyed competing against herself and getting her handicap down to twenty-eight.

Now living in Paris, the opportunity to exercise is limited. So what does she do? She walks – whether it's picking Lois up from school, going to L'Alliance Française or whatever. Naomi doesn't exercise by running round in circles like I do. She has always undertaken activities when the opportunities presented themselves, and from the comfortable distance of my word processor I would venture to say that, maybe to Naomi, walking to pick up her daughter from school is every bit as rewarding an activity as single-handedly circumnavigating the globe.

Naomi James single-handedly sailed round the world and now walks to keep fit

Desmond Lynam

Des started a love affair with sport as a lanky teenager at a grammar school in Sussex. Thirty years later, the affair is still going strong and, as presenter of BBC Television's sports programmes, he is in the enviable position of doing what he loves most, combining his passion for sport with journalism.

Now aged forty-eight, with his weight stable at 180 lbs, Des has been 6 ft 1½ ins tall since he was fourteen years old, having shot up earlier than usual to his adult height. Weighing only 126 lbs, he started to box which his father encouraged because he said, 'You'll get over your fear and people will respect you for having the courage to do it.' But, although he appreciated the skill factor, his fear of being knocked out put Des off and he was never comfortable with it. 'Best laxative known to man!' He still has a fascination with the skill aspect and for many years has been the BBC Radio boxing commentator.

As a schoolboy, Des was a good all-round soccer player and a useful, medium-paced bowler before he gave up cricket to play tennis. 'In those days, you taught yourself. I used to watch Lew Hoad on the telly and play in the park. I played for my school. It's the one sport where if someone had got hold of me I think I could have done something.' He still enjoys playing, and each June is able to indulge his pleasure vicariously from the commentary box at Wimbledon.

Apart from a couple of episodes of rampant bachelorhood, when take-aways and rubbish food were staples, Des has always eaten well. He loves pasta of all kinds and anything

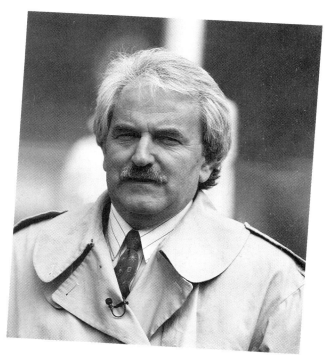

Desmond Lynam, well-known face of BBC sport

Italian like sardines and olive oil. He occasionally enjoys a steak but otherwise has cut down on red meat. Aware of the cholesterol-lowering effects of oats, every day starts with a bowl of home-made porridge made with water, not milk, and a little sugar plus a banana or two. His real weakness is a sweet tooth, especially for ice cream – Italian naturally.

Social drinking is part of the job and in the past an occasional 'session with the boys' was not unheard of. But Des now limits his intake to about twenty units a week in the form of good wine, Scotch whisky and sometimes vodka. He recently went off alcohol completely for three months. 'Felt absolutely fine but no good socially – dull so-and-so. I never like drinking at lunchtime either – it's fun for an hour and then I go right down.'

Des has never smoked even though both his parents did. 'Even as a little kid I thought it was stupid. But if my friends want to smoke in my house I would never stop them. I don't like to see young people smoking though, especially young girls – it seems so pointless.'

Des's current exercise routine

Des's daily exercise routine consists of twenty sit-ups ('couldn't bear the stomach to go') and about 400 running-on-the-spot (for aerobic fitness) which takes no more than fifteen minutes. He plays golf twice a week to a handicap of fifteen. Minus a dog, Des takes himself for a mile walk each day and, when on holiday in the sun, will spend hours swimming in the sea.

At one point, he went to a gym three times a week for six months and became quite obsessive about it but, ironically, he never felt worse physically, having constant colds and feeling wretchedly tired. It obviously didn't suit him.

In fact, a less obsessional person than Des you are unlikely to meet and, although he does admit to a certain self-absorption about his health in general, his attitude to diet and exercise is one of informed moderation – relaxed and with a strong dash of humour – just what you'd expect really.

Geoff Hurst

Life has never been the same for Geoff since that memorable day in July 1966 when England beat West Germany 4-2 to win the World Cup at Wembley. The millions that watched that magnificent game will never forget Geoff's hat-trick, two of the goals scored in extra time, the other goal scored by Martin Peters, Geoff's West Ham teammate. Even now, never a day passes without someone reminding him of that event. 'People remember exactly where they were and what they were doing at the time – people who were only maybe aged 10 remember clearly about that game. It was a great day for the country. It transcends sport when you get that far.'

Having kicked a ball around since he could walk, Geoff first joined West Ham as an apprentice ground staff player at age seventeen in 1958. It wasn't long before he proved his outstanding ability and was signed as a professional the following year. In those early days, he was equally talented at cricket and in 1962 he played for Essex. But, unable to play both games professionally, he chose soccer as his career. Geoff spent nearly thirty years playing football and later managing clubs, including Chelsea from 1979-1981. The first fourteen were spent playing for his 'alma mater', West Ham, during the golden age of the club when they won the FA Cup in 1964. Following the World Cup, he gained 49 England caps between 1966 and 1972.

Geoff always found it a joy to be fit. Although the work was very strenuous, it was a pleasure to train and play the game he loved so much, and to be paid for doing it. 'I was a

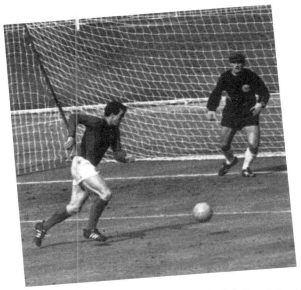

Geoff Hurst in the 1966 World Cup Final

and, having left the days of the post-match drink behind, nowadays enjoys dry white wine with a meal. Although his time is at a premium, Geoff wants to spend more of it playing sport and is considering joining his daughter on the tennis court. Fitness for fitness' sake is not enough to sustain him in sticking to an exercise routine. Like me, he needs the challenge of a game which requires a skill to be developed. With his outstanding natural sporting talent, he has got it made.

totally dedicated professional – my whole mind and body were geared towards playing and turning out for the game on Saturday. To reach the top you have to have that kind of obsessiveness to be successful.' Although he stopped playing professionally in 1979, aged thirty-nine, he stayed pretty active until 1986 playing in charity matches, in particular for Dennis Waterman's Showbiz team.

Geoff's current exercise routine

Now aged fifty, weighing 204 lbs (just over a stone heavier than his playing weight) and 6 ft tall, Geoff looks fit and feels very well. He plays golf in the summer and recently took part in a 7-side tournament in Singapore demonstrating that his skill endures even though he is no longer at peak fitness. He has always eaten well and sensibly, never smoked

Bobby Moore

The most unforgettable image many people have of Bobby was when, as England captain, he received the World Cup trophy at Wembley in 1966. Although that momentous occasion was certainly the high point, Bobby's football career was long and distinguished. He joined West Ham United at seventeen in the same year as Geoff Hurst and both were signed as professionals within a few months in 1958. Also like Geoff, Bobby was a gifted cricketer. As a schoolboy, he was initially more successful in this sport, playing for Essex Boys, London Boys and England Boys – a level he didn't quite reach in soccer at the time. He made up for it later in aces, though, when he was picked to play for England 108 times (a record that has only recently been surpassed by Peter Shilton) including three World Cups: Chile 1962, and Mexico 1970, as well as England 1966. It is his reputation as England captain that is unmatched, having led the England side on 90 occasions. He also

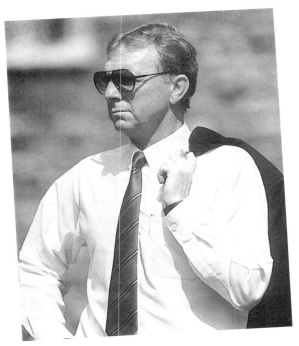

Bobby Moore exercises regularly to stay fit

captained West Ham to their FA Cup win in 1964 and the European Cup Winners' Cup in 1965. This is some achievement but when I asked Bobby what special qualities he must have had to receive these accolades, he replied, 'I don't know, but I do know what my weak spots are. What's important is to have the right attitude and the right application. Give one hundred per cent in everything you do – you cannot do more than that.'

Was there a key element in the spectacular success of the England team and some top clubs in the mid-60s? 'There was a real continuity in players, staff and management; clubs were able to balance the books and there was not a great deal of financial difference in playing for one team or another. So players

tended to stay put with one club. The situation was stable and the continuity resulted in a consistency in the game that I believe was an important contributing factor to our success both at club and international level.'

Bobby stopped playing professionally in the 1980s after a stint at Fulham and some very enjoyable years in which he combined football and travel, playing in North America, Australia and South Africa.

Bobby's current exercise routine

Now aged fifty, Bobby maintains a constant level of fitness; four or five times a week, he runs for 25 minutes on the heath near his home with the dog, or he skips with a rope and rounds it off with a few abdominal exercises. He plays squash for pleasure, if time allows, about three times a week in the winter. But he loves to get out in the fresh air as much as possible so he plays golf and tennis in the summer – sports that were not available to him as a schoolboy. At 6 ft tall and 175 lbs in weight – a few pounds lighter than when playing – Bobby's diet contains no red meat, very little dairy produce or animal fats, but plenty of fish, chicken, fresh fruit and vegetables. After having abdominal surgery earlier this year, he made a few dietary alterations but the pleasure he derives from eating has not been blunted. He has never smoked, and drinks beer and wine, socially.

Bobby is still deeply involved in the game of soccer, commenting on games three times a week for Capital Gold radio. Although not fanatical about fitness, he has always exercised and, one suspects, he always will.

TEN

Achieving the Targets

Liz's story

East Grinstead remains unvisited, still just a name on the map halfway between Crawley and Royal Tunbridge Wells. I did not make it to the short-course triathlon held there, or indeed anywhere. But in the course of failing to achieve that particular goal I discovered a lot about what motivates me and, more generally, how individual is the business of motivation.

Andy was right when he said at the beginning of this book that one of the benefits that come with age is a decreasing need to chase rainbows. Competing in a triathlon is a particular rainbow that I can certainly forego. All physical exercise is work and the triathlon is harder work than almost any other. I suspect I am a trifle too lazy to engage in the triple excesses of the swim-bike-run regime but I prefer to believe, like Robert Louis Stevenson, that 'a faculty for idleness implies a catholic appetite and a strong sense of personal identity'.

Being fairly hedonistic, I need more pleasure, enjoyment and fun mixed in with the effort than seems possible when slogging it out training in three excessively physically demanding disciplines. Andy exercises because he enjoys it for its own sake. I have a friend like Andy who, when he goes on holiday, starts his day with a 20-mile cycle ride, follows that up with a swim before lunch and fills the afternoon with an hour or so of running. He does it because he loves the feel of using his body and muscles. I too like the experience of physical activity but for me the challenge is in acquiring a skill in the process which is why I chose a skill-based sport like diving. Physical fitness was almost a by-product that was the result of endless repetitions, jumping off springboards in all manner of contortions, to achieve consistency – which is what wins medals – and, ultimately, perfection.

People like Andy and my friend, Philip, are very disciplined about their training. They set themselves specific physical goals and targets and get a kick out of achieving them. I am less concerned with the experience of exercising my muscles and more with the sense of elation when a specific movement comes together and is experienced as near to perfect as one could hope for.

So, I have discovered why I love to ski and why, recently, after relegating my ancient wooden tennis racket to the attic along with other bits of antique sporting ephemera and replacing it with a new, lightweight graphite job, I proceeded to enjoy a summer of discovery of drop shots, half volleys and top spin under the expert tutelage of Russell Bolton in North Oxford. What joy on those rare occasions when everything seemed to go just right – the timing, the rhythm, the thwack of the ball on the racket, the ball placed perfectly just out of Russell's reach. The sensation was one of flowing, with ease and grace, effortlessly.

When I was a child I was chided for lolling in chairs the wrong way round with my head where my feet should have been and vice versa, and with being clumsy. I have been searching ever since for ways to overcome this apparent deficiency and to emerge as the graceful swan. When I mis-hit the tennis ball, I grunt and growl and jump up and down with frustration; but, oh, what bliss when I get it right. And, as soon as it's done, it's gone and there is the next ball to play. Bonk, the ball hits the frame and out it sails into the car park.

The great thing about aiming for perfection is that, even while you're thinking you've got it, it's gone and there you are still trying. It isn't the goal that's important but the process of trying to achieve it. Abraham Maslow, the American humanistic psychologist, called those instances of real excellence, of real perfection, 'peak experiences'. Apparently most people, at some time or another, have peak experiences – just think of the single, most blissful, joyous moment of your whole life, a truly unmistakable experience. The effect on the body of this kind of stimulation is to tickle up our feelings, emotions, autonomic nervous system and hormones.

Another American psychologist, Mikaly Csikszentmihalyi, called these feelings 'optimal experiences'. He interviewed people from all walks of life, including artists, athletes, composers, dancers and scientists, and found that when they described how it feels when they are doing something that is worth doing for its own sake, many used the word 'flow'. He says that, 'To remain in flow, one needs to increase the complexity of the activity by developing new skills and taking on new challenges. This holds just as true for enjoying business, playing the piano, or enjoying playing with the children, as for the game of tennis . . . Flow forces people to stretch themselves, to take on another challenge, to improve on their abilities.'

It seems apparent to me that this quality of flow so typical of clearly structured activities, like sports and games, is an important motivator. Since the level of challenges and skills

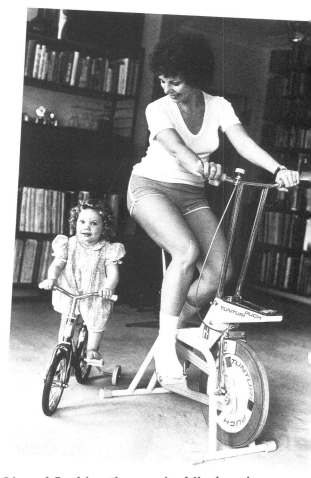

Liz and Sophie – the exercise bike has since been abandoned in favour of tennis and golf

can be varied and controlled, everyone can have this kind of optimal experience whether you are an absolute beginner or an Olympic champion.

In 1991, a tome entitled *Exercise, Fitness and Health – A Consensus of Current Knowledge* was published with contributions from the most eminent scientists in the field. Concerning motivation, the consensus was that knowledge and information about the relationship of exercise, fitness and health, together with attitudes and beliefs about the benefits, are all helpful in making the decision to adopt a more active lifestyle. But the problem is in maintaining and adhering to an exercise programme. The advice offered was to focus on specific incentives for the individual with concrete rewards such as enjoyment and personal satisfaction.

So at last I have discovered why I find riding the stationary bike at home so difficult to keep up no matter how convenient. I need the challenge of improving a skill. In addition to my new-found interest in tennis, a little late I admit, I plan to take up golf which seems the perfect activity – a constant challenge impossible to achieve! On a daily basis, there are always the dogs, Bebe, Cleo and Domie to take me for walks. I hope that now they realize the good it is doing me, they won't find it *quite* such a chore.

Andy's Story

Remember the principles set out in Chapter 2 – set a target plan, write it out, do it, record it. Well, here's how I got on with my aim of taking up five new activities.

Sailing

I've never done much, if any, sailing before, but I've always had the usual clichéd, born-at-arms-length, romantic idea about the sea. My father, who spent fifty odd (probably very odd) years as a merchant seaman, couldn't stand the sea. So my latent interest must have come from my own naivety and my mum.

So, in the interests of all old men, last year I bought an Enterprise dinghy for £400 through the ads in the local paper, joined Weir Wood Sailing Club in deepest East Sussex, enrolled at The City of London Polytechnic Yachtmaster's night-school course and took two three-day dinghy-sailing courses at Emsworth Sailing School near Chichester.

Dinghy sailing

First, buy a wet suit. Second, there is a big difference between sailing on a reservoir and on tidal water. This may sound obvious but tidal-water dinghy sailing is dangerous and you really should know what you're doing. Reservoir sailing, by comparison, is a doddle, although not without its dangers. Reservoir sailors spend most of their time racing around buoys and shouting at each other, while tidal dinghy sailors agonize over currents and tides and then live life in the fast stream. Both types get wet.

I like dinghy sailing on warm days with between a force 2–3 wind blowing, preferably in a dinghy hired by the hour in a warm tideless sea. Real dinghy sailors do it at dusk in the Bristol Channel in January. Not for me, thanks.

Cruiser sailing

Having spent a year completing the land-based Yachtmaster course, eight of us (five men, three women) decided to try out our new skills. So at the end of the course we hired out a Sun Kiss 40 in Falmouth for ten days.

We had a mixture of backgrounds and abilities, which seemed to blend quite well. The Thames lighterman was just terrific at controlling the boat under power in the marina which is the place most yachting accidents occur. We had a navigator who should have been born in the sixteenth century and a couple of dinghy sailors who knew all about setting sails. The rest of us were sick most of the time.

There is no privacy on a forty-foot boat, particularly as regards bowel movements. Once you get over this novel experience, which you do quite quickly, everything else, eating badly, being sick (not always in that order), not sleeping, being scared witless, dying of boredom, all soon fall into place.

We headed west, with an unusual light April easterly wind, to the Scilly Isles, anchoring in New Grimsby on the Tresco side; as the wind changed to come from the more familiar south-westerly direction, we sailed due east to Guernsey in the Channel Islands, then headed south to Treguerier on the north coast of France and hopped back across the channel to Portsmouth and down the coast to Falmouth. I feel rather proud writing that and we all had a sense of achievement, but April still can get a bit windy, and round-the-world yachtspeople have my unreserved admiration for their ability to withstand long periods of boredom interspersed with moments of utter fear.

So, like my dad, I'm only a fair-weather sailor, although I must have enjoyed it as I've agreed to join a pal who is going to sail around Britain next June.

Distance swimming

This may seem to follow on naturally from sailing, but it doesn't. All my swimming, with the exception of the swim leg of the Alderney and the English Riviera (Torquay to you and me) triathlons, has been in the comparative chlorinated comfort of local authority swimming pools.

My initial interest in swimming grew out of the TV 'Superstars' competition and then, more recently, out of triathlon training. In a short-course triathlon you swim 1.5 kilometres, which is sixty lengths of a standard pool. In an open-water swim the distance varies but is usually about a mile, unless the water temperature is 11°C or less when, under the British Triathlon Association rules, they can reduce the distance.

Indoor swimming

Swimming in a pool is non-threatening, other than the chlorine which probably doesn't do your hair, eyes, skin, etc. much good. However, you can follow the black line and count the lengths. You know where you are. The water may limit your sense of smell, taste, hearing and sight (although not your sense of touch) but it is weight-supporting and is said to be, and probably is, the best way of taking exercise. It's kind on your joints. Once you can swim five lengths and you get into a rhythm and get your breathing right it doesn't take too long to continue swimming until boredom becomes the limiting factor.

Out of curiosity I swam five kilometres (200 lengths) in the Newhaven Leisure Pool as part of the British Sports Association for the Disabled 1991 Swimathon. It took me 2 hours, 11 minutes. Now that isn't particularly quick but, apart from the tedium, I can't think of any other exercise, walking included, from which I experienced such little muscular/joint reaction for such a period of cardiovascular endurance. Swimming does seem to be the kindest exercise of all on the body and twenty minutes a day is an excellent way of exercising, provided you can put up with the chlorine, ennui and changing facilities. Now sprint training and swimming in the open sea are something else.

Open-water swimming

For a novice like me open-water sea swims in UK tidal waters are disorientating. The water temperature around Alderney in early June was 13°C. It was a 1500-metre swim and everyone wore a wet suit, which floats you out of the water, making you more buoyant but less familiar with the environment. Now 750 metres in a straight line is a long way and in a massed start it's every man/woman for themselves. I couldn't see, someone knocked my goggles off, my lungs expanded as I swam and my wet suit got increasingly restrictive. I lost sense of time, distance and direction; the diesel fumes from the rescue boat hung over the water. And, wet suit or not, 13°C is cold. In a swimming pool the average speed is about two miles an hour. In the sea, drift and currents, even at slack water, change your position, but then again, as I mentioned above, it's hard to know where you are or where you're going anyway. The forty minutes it took me to

complete the 750 metres should ensure I don't do too many UK tidal-water swims. Mr Panic and I were not too far apart. On the other hand I love swimming in the warm, tideless, polluted but clear Mediterranean.

Sprint training is for fifteen-year-olds at 7.00 a.m. in the local pool, five days a week.

Golf

'It's a great game. Starting in your mid-forties is a bit late, but as you're a sportsman you should be able to take it up, no trouble,' said the golf professional at Holtye Golf Club.

I didn't explain that, although I was grateful for any compliments, his accolade to me as a sportsman was based on the fact that once I could run quickly which, as far as I can tell, is not a prime requirement for a golfer. As a ball player I've always been found wanting. I have played golf on average about three times a year for the last ten years. However, here's the paradox: because I say yes to most opportunities and because people need ageing micro-celebrities who like a day out, I have been invited to, and played (could be the wrong verb), on some of what are reputed to be the finest golf courses in the land. I don't get invited back very often, although I'm pretty good at lunch and I do try very hard.

If you turn up at the Bernard Cribbins Golf Classic without any clubs, because you haven't got any, the assumption is that you are yet another ageing sportsman hiding his light under a bushel. The expression on a golf course seems to be 'a bandit' – which I believe is someone who used to have a handicap of, say, fifteen but can now be technically correct in declaring twenty-four, and proceeds to snitch all the silverware. This is something I would like to do but I haven't got the ability and, as handicaps start at twenty-four and I've never scored under 105, it's all fairly hypothetical. Good old Bernard; he keeps asking me back.

I have, of course, been seduced by that shot you make every so often that you get as right as a well-done sum. I also do potter down to a driving range to whang a basket of balls about; this takes about half an hour as opposed to the half a day that a full round takes.

I have, however, learnt one thing. By and large, other than your partner, to whom you'll have to be extra nice, people really don't mind you being useless, provided you a) obey all the rules, b) enjoy yourself but, most importantly, c) you don't lose your ball. Having to look for the ball of a player who averages eight shots a hole is apparently deadly. So you need a nice little 3-iron shot that goes straight for about seventy-five yards and, while everyone's not necessarily happy, they'll put up with you for the next three-and-a-half hours and regard it as some sort of missionary work. I think I could like golf, but not yet. Not while there are trainers to be worn out.

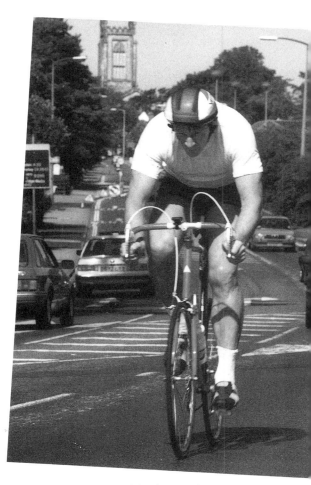

Andy's most enjoyable form of exercise

10-mile pursuit cycling

This might not seem like the ideal sport for a forty-plus-year-old to take up. But it's something I've been twiddling with ever since I gave up rugby two years ago.

Cycling is dangerous in that motorized road users often disregard or just don't see cyclists and you can get blown away. Also, simply falling off a bike isn't exactly a barrel-load of laughs.

However, for me, cycling has become the most enjoyable form of exercise. It's weight-supporting, you get to see places and people, it's demanding of your cardiovascular system and you can still compete. What's more, if you can cycle to work/play then not only are you exercising but there's a reason for the activity. The main drawback, at least for me, is that you are limited in that, between late October and late March, it's dark and the weather is, as they say, usually inclement. As a spring to autumn activity it's great.

As cycling is one of the three disciplines of the triathlon (swimming and running being the other two), in order to get some advice I joined East Grinstead Cycling Club. Every Wednesday evening in the summer they hold a 10-mile pursuit competition. I turned up on my old £50 bike, bought fifteen years ago, in a pair of trainers and old shorts. Again, like the golf club, they assumed I must be brilliant or a complete dork. I was not brilliant. Cycling clubs are high fashion centres; you, quite frankly, would not believe the money fifteen-year-olds will spend on the right pair of shades.

The majority of cyclists are under twenty or over thirty-five but they tend to dress the same: bright (to be seen) and tight (less wind resistance). They have the same body shape, similar to a distance runner. The good news is that, unlike distance running, provided you don't go up too many hills you can get away with weighing 245 lbs, given that you can afford the repair and maintenance bills on the bike.

As ever, the real competition is against your own past performances. So if you start from a low base you can see yourself improve and you can help that process by buying the right kit. I now have a twenty-seven-inch, bespoke Allin frame bike, with the slot-in cycle shoes, aero bars, Fagor cycle vest and pants and I've seen a very nice pair of Bolle shades. I'm still a

dork but I look the part and it's twenty-five minutes of real heart, lungs and leg effort. Also, the nice thing about cycling is that it's a club activity and attracts all ages, backgrounds, male and female and if you haven't been on a warm summer Sunday morning club run over Ashdown Forest before the cars get up, then do go and do it. What's more, there seem to be a load of guys much older than me still biking, appearing to enjoy themselves and taking some serious exercise without giving their bodies too much of a pounding.

The health club

Health club is a label, like hotel, that covers a very broad church (yet another label) that also defies generalizations.

The basis of most private or public health clubs is that you pay a fee (which varies enormously), for facilities (which vary enormously), for the use of those facilities for a period of time ranging from not very long to forever.

I must here declare a personal interest. I was a member of Cannon's Club in London for eight years, Chairman of the Barbican Club for a couple of years and now have an interest in the Espree Club at the Royal Mint.

What I've found is that there tends to be no common thread linking people's reasons for joining these clubs. The reasons vary, the strangest and surprisingly common one being that, by paying a cheque, the financial pain eases the guilt amassed through not taking exercise. More usefully, the club may be handy to get to from work or home and can also be used as a base to jog from. Both women and men sometimes feel vulnerable for whatever reason about their body shape and find a health-club atmosphere non-threatening and protective. Some clubs offer special classes in yoga, tai chi and karate so it can become a mental as well as a physical work-out. But most people join for a fitness programme based around exercise classes (aerobics) or the machines. The machines fall into two main categories, weights or cardiovascular.

Weights can either be free weights, which need experience in handling, or weights locked into a machine (fixed); Nautilus, Cybex, Keiser are some of the leading makes. Each machine will have a graded resistance and will focus on a particular set of muscles; it is not only advisable but necessary to get tuition in using weights, even when fixed. I personally have never been particularly interested in either fixed or free weights but it is a way of building or toning muscles, changing your shape and building power.

Cardiovascular machines for exercising the heart and lungs are usually the most used equipment in any club. They take the form of cycling machines, treadmills, stair/step machines, rowing machines, upper body exercisers. There is something about using these machines that reminds you about hamsters on a wheel in a cage. To counteract this and to encourage you to use them as part of a regular fitness programme, the manufacturers include all sorts of anti-boredom devices, from giving instant and recorded feedback, such as heart rate, speed, resistance, distance 'travelled' and time, to TV screens and videos.

Personally, I'm a fan of health clubs provided you use them on your own terms. There is undoubtedly an element of the work ethic associated with these clubs: 'Working to get fit,' 'The best investment you can make is in your own body,' etc., etc. Some people enjoy that aspect, others find it a turn-off. However, if you are not well motivated but feel you want to do some exercise which is appropriate for you, whatever your real or perceived limitations, and to get some advice, guidance and a word of encouragement, then (at a price) health clubs offer the discipline of a regular exercise routine.

Trite but right summary

The conclusion I've reached after trying and semi-participating in these activities – other than 'variety is the spice of life' – is that you have to enjoy what you're doing and the company you're keeping. Otherwise, it's a chore and at forty-plus there are too many enjoyable fitness activities, whatever your physical limitations, to continue with those that are perceived by you as being a bit of a drudge.

Index